NATURAL HEALING WITH QIGONG

NATURAL HEALING WITH QIGONG

THERAPEUTIC QIGONG

DR. AIHAN KUHN CMD.

YMAA Publication Center
Wolfeboro, NH USA

YMAA Publication Center, Inc.
Main Office
PO Box 480 Washington Street
Wolfeboro, N.H. 03894
1-800-669-8892 • www.ymaa.com • info@ymaa.com

20200505

Editor: Susan Bullowa
Cover Design: Richard Rossiter

Anatomy drawing page 88 provided by are used by permission from the LifeART Collection of Images © 1989-1997 by Techpool Studios, Cleveland, OH.

Publisher's Cataloging in Publication

Kuhn, Aihan.

Natural healing with Qigong : therapeutic Qigong / Aihan Kuhn. --
1st ed. -- Boston, Mass. : YMAA Publication Center, 2004.

p. ; cm.

Includes bibliographical references and index.
ISBN: 1-59439-001-0

1. Qi gong. 2. Medicine, Chinese. 3. Holistic medicine. 4. Mind
and body. I. Title.

RA781.8 .K86 2004   2004106334
613.7/148--dc22   0405

Disclaimer:
The author and publisher of this material are NOT RESPONSIBLE in any manner whatsoever for any injury which may occur through reading or following the instructions in this manual. The activities, physical or otherwise, described in this material may be too strenuous or dangerous for some people, and the reader(s) should consult a physician before engaging in them.

This book is only intended to assist with healing and disease prevention and is not meant to be a substitute for any medication or the advice of your physician. Please consult with your doctor if you have severe illness.

Printed in USA.

Table of Contents

Dedication

I dedicate this book to my cousin Zhu Hong who first introduced me to this particular Qigong exercise. She was the person who opened the door for me in 1976. It is also dedicated to my teachers: Grand Masters Feng Zhi Qiang and Duan Zhi Liang.

I never believed in Qigong before. I didn't even believe in Traditional Chinese Medicine. In 1978 Zhu Hong told me about these exercises; I tried them and felt improvement in my health almost immediately. That is when I decided to study Qigong.

Grand Master Feng Zhi Qiang is one of the most famous Chen style Taiji masters in China. Grand Master Duan Zhi Liang is one of the most famous Qigong masters. Both of them have had a tremendous influence on my practice, my teaching, my healing methods, and my life.

Dr. Aihan Kuhn,
CMD, DIPL. ABT

Romanization of Chinese Words

This book primarily uses the Pinyin romanization system of Chinese to English. Pinyin is standard in the People's Republic of China, and in several world organizations, including the United Nations. Pinyin, which was introduced in China in the 1950's, replaces the Wade-Giles and Yale systems. In some cases, the more popular spelling of a word may be used for clarity.

Some common conversions:

Pinyin	Also Spelled As	Pronunciation
Qi	Chi	chē
Qigong	Chi Kung	chē kŭng
Qin Na	Chin Na	chǐn nă
Jin	Jing	jǐn
Gongfu	Kung Fu	gŏng foo
Taijiquan	Tai Chi Chuan	tī jē chüén

For more information, please refer to *The People's Republic of China: Administrative Atlas, The Reform of the Chinese Written Language,* or a contemporary manual of style.

The author and publisher have taken the liberty of not italicizing words of foreign origin in this text. This decision was made to make the text easier to read. Please see the comprehensive glossary for definitions of Chinese words.

Preface—My Path to Natural Medicine

By Aihan Kuhn

When I was in medical school in China studying conventional Western medicine, I did not believe in Traditional Chinese Medicine (TCM) and Qigong. I thought, "Qigong" was "Cheat Gong" and was completely superstitious. I thought Chinese medicine was just "comfort therapy" and not real medicine. In China, all the medical schools were required to teach TCM, and all of the medical students were required to study TCM. Therefore, I had to memorize the content, including the theory of Yin Yang, Five Elements, Zhang Fu, Jin, Qi, Shen, physical examination of Glossy tongue, Slippery pulse, and therapeutic methods using herbs, acupuncture points, and meridians. The hardest part to study was TCM theory. At that time, I was 24 years old. I had no idea what Qi was. How can you identify or measure Qi? Who could understand the Chinese Kidney or Chinese Liver? I was completely skeptical. I just wanted to memorize the textbook and pass the test with a good score and that was all. I did well on my tests; I received a 91 on my final test on TCM. Nevertheless, the truth was, I really did not have a deep understanding. Even after I graduated from Hunan Medical University, I still did not believe that TCM was real medicine.

Soon after I began working in the hospital, I had a severe toothache. It was a kind of nerve pain. I could not sleep at night due to the pain, even with pain medication and antibiotics. At this point, I was ready to try anything to relieve the pain. I got up and went to an acupuncture doctor. (In China, we do not say acupuncturist, we say acupuncture doctor because they study medicine for five years in medical school). He used three needles, two on my face and one on my hand. Fifteen minutes later the pain was reduced by 80%. To me, that was a miracle because I had taken several pain medications and had not gotten relief. Now, I was so happy that I could finally sleep.

Some time later, I had my first child and started breastfeeding. One month later, I developed an infection at the nipple. I took an antibiotic for several days and was using a topical antibiotic cream. The infection was not going away and I was experiencing intolerable pain that was affecting my breast-feeding. My milk production was now also diminished, and my poor baby was crying because she was hungry. She hated the cow's milk that I was substituting for her. I decided to go the obstetrics and gynecology department of a TCM hospital where a doctor looked at my problem. She did not give me a prescription of herbs. Instead, she suggested that I wash the area with rice water everyday, 3 or 4 times a day. In China, we always had to wash the rice before cooking it, so that was the rice water to which she was referring. I was really expecting some miracle herbs, but I followed her instructions anyway. On the second day, the pain was reduced; on the third day, the infection was more than 50% improved and the pain had subsided.

On the fourth and fifth days, I felt almost normal with very little discomfort. I could not believe it. I thought that using an antibiotic for infection was the correct thing to do because this was what we had learned in school. I went back to the doctor and asked her why the rice water was so effective. She explained that the rice water contains much B vitamins, especially B1. The skin will dry and crack from a lack of B vitamins. By supplying nutrition to the area, the skin was able to heal quickly. What a lesson I had learned. I had not learned about rice water in medical school.

After several similar experiences, I started to believe in the power of TCM and natural healing. It all made sense. I began to realize that because we came from nature, nature is really a vast and beneficial resource for us to use. I remember one time when I was in the countryside, a farmer had told me: "Anything growing that is green might be a medicine, only we have not found a use for it yet." It was then that I decided to use Chinese medicine in my practice. I began to use acupuncture and Chinese herbal medicine in my obstetrics and gynecology practice. My patients responded very well with Chinese medicine.

After living in the United States for a while, I began to have back pain, insomnia, asthma, chronic sinus problems, headaches, hip problems, and wrist tendonitis. I am totally fine now thanks to Chinese medicine, except for a little "over-worked syndrome" that I need to pay more attention to in balancing my life in the future. I teach and practice Taiji, Qigong and other Chinese healing exercises regularly. I use them for my own healing as well as to maintain my energy level and immune function. I explain Tai Chi and Qigong to my students from a medical point of view, stating how this type of exercise can help to assist healing and disease prevention. Many students have recovered from their physical, mental, and emotional ailments. I have created a

	WOOD 木	FIRE 火	EARTH 土	METAL 金	WATER 水
DIRECTION	EAST	SOUTH	CENTER	WEST	NORTH
SEASON	SPRING	SUMMER	LONG SUMMER	AUTUMN	WINTER
CLIMACTIC CONDITION	WIND	SUMMER HEAT	DAMPNESS	DRYNESS	COLD
PROCESS	BIRTH	GROWTH	TRANSFORMATION	HARVEST	STORAGE
COLOR	GREEN	RED	YELLOW	WHITE	BLACK
TASTE	SOUR	BITTER	SWEET	PUNGENT	SALTY
SMELL	GOATISH	BURNING	FRAGRANT	RANK	ROTTEN
YIN ORGAN	LIVER	HEART	SPLEEN	LUNGS	KIDNEYS
YANG ORGAN	GALL BLADDER	SMALL INTESTINE	STOMACH	LARGE INTESTINE	BLADDER
OPENING	EYES	TONGUE	MOUTH	NOSE	EARS
TISSUE	SINEWS	BLOOD VESSELS	FLESH	SKIN/HAIR	BONES
EMOTION	ANGER	HAPPINESS	PENSIVENESS	SADNESS	FEAR
HUMAN SOUND	SHOUT	LAUGHTER	SONG	WEEPING	GROAN

TABLE OF CORRESPONDENCES ASSOCIATED WITH THE FIVE PHASES

harmonious and joyful environment in my clinic so that people feel good just being there. I use Chinese medicine to treat all kinds of problems. The results are incredible and sometimes even I am astonished, but I know it is not only from my years of experience in medicine but also from knowing how to apply the Qi in each treatment.

Qigong is an excellent preventative medicine. My father had tuberculosis beginning at 9 years of age that lasted through the wartime. After the liberation of People's Republic of China in 1949, he was treated and got better, but he always had a poor foundation for his health. He later developed COPD and cancer. He died several years ago. His genes passed to me, so I carry his gene for poor lung energy. My mother had severe arthritis since she was forty. I also carry her gene for poor kidney energy. Their illnesses pushed me to practice natural medicine for myself because I do not want to end up in the same condition as they did. So far, I am much better off than the average person is my age. I use Qigong and Taiji to prevent illness. As long as I continue to practice, I do not need to worry about health issues.

In school, I never knew that TCM could do so much for people. I suggest that everyone should try Chinese medicine to experience its benefits. Without having tried it, I would still not believe in TCM. After trying it, it has made a big difference in my practice, my life, my health, my energy, as well as my family's health.

In 1995, I went back to China to continue my education in TCM, Taiji and Qigong. I worked in a TCM hospital and rotated in the Department of Acupuncture, Chinese Massage, TCM Dermatology, and TCM Orthopedics. After regular work in the hospital, I continued my study of Qigong, Taiji, and other Martial Arts. I spent 12 hours a day studying and working. I had an excellent teacher in TCM. I learned so much TCM theory and hands-on therapy. This experience opened my eyes as well as my heart to the path of TCM.

The lack of attention and support from the government contributed to the low self-esteem of some TCM practitioners. They had to be convinced that Chinese medicine is a treasure from our ancestors—gift to our society from ancient China. It is the most complete natural healing system and has tremendous value. Chinese medicine holds 4000 years of value due to its safety and minimal side effects. It is highly efficient for treating many illnesses. It supports the mind-body connection and yields long-term benefits. Even though lacking in support from the government, the TCM practitioner should continue to perform this wonderful natural healing art.

Chinese medicine and Qigong exercises are a wonderful approach to natural healing. They have helped me to improve my body and my mind. Even my memory has improved. They can help many ailments, but not everything. The healing effect depends on the severity and the duration of the illness, the patient's cooperation, life style, diet, exercise habits, and mindset, as well as other factors. The closer you are to nature, and are open minded, and disciplined, you can expect good results. The more drugs you take, the less healthy you are; the more stubborn you are and unwilling to change, the less healthy you will be both mentally and physically. The more regularly you practice Qigong, the less you will need to see the doctor.

You can practice Qigong regularly for a year to see what happens in your life. If you still feel the same after a year, you can say Qigong does not work. I hope this book will give you enough information to open the door for you to this wonderful ancient Chinese Healing art and human energy science.

Dr. Aihan Kuhn,
CMD, DIPL. ABT

Acknowledgements

It is not hard for me to express my Qigong knowledge but it is difficult for a Chinese-speaking person like me to write a book in English. It took a great deal of time and effort to figure out how to say things right, how to put the language into the right order and make good sentences. In Chinese, we speak and write in the opposite order from English, so we say "English speaks opposite". On the other hand, an English speaker could say we speak opposite. To finish this book, I needed much help. Therefore, I would like to take this opportunity to thank all the people who reviewed this book, made many corrections for me, and gave me so much encouragement.

I'd like to thank Gerry Kuhn, my dear husband who did the first edit. He is the one who had to try to translate my Chinglish into English. I cannot imagine how much he had to put up with my first draft. I would like to thank Professor Jean Lacey from Babson College who did further language corrections, and who gave me some valuable suggestions. I would like to thank Dr. Kenneth Sancier from The Qigong Institute who also gave me professional suggestions and encouragement. Finally, I would like to thank Professor Matthew Nichol from Berkley College, who did more editing and corrections on this book. Their time, effort, and their encouragement are greatly appreciated. I do not think I could have accomplished this project without their help.

I would also like to thank to all of my students who are dedicated to the study of Qigong and Taiji. Their dedication motivates me to continue to explore the power of Qigong. Improvements in their general well-being and health have given me more confidence, both in teaching and exploring. Their compliments gave me strength to "fight" with close-minded Western trained medical practitioners. They have helped to prove my belief that if you work hard on natural healing, the healing will happen.

I want to thank all of the instructors trained at CMH (Chinese Medicine for Health), and who have been teaching at CMH for many years. They help me to maintain a tradition of high quality by teaching and spreading the knowledge of the energy medicine. Their hard work is greatly appreciated.

I want to thank the board members of TQHI (Tai Chi & Qi Gong Healing Institute, a non-profit institute established in 1998), who put their time and energy into promoting Qigong Healing as well as organizing the World Tai Chi and Qigong Day in Massachusetts every year. Their hard work has had a remarkable effect in our community.

I thank my mentor, Grand Master Feng Zhi Qiang, a very well known grand master of Chen style Taijiquan in China, who taught me the fundamental principles of Chen style Taiji practice. I also want to thank Duan Zhi Liang, another very well known Qigong master in China, who not only taught me Qigong, but also taught me how to apply Qigong to achieve a stress-free and quality lifestyle. They have given me much valuable information regarding Qigong and Taiji practice.

I thank all Qigong practitioners and instructors who maintain their faith in this ancient energy medicine, help to spread the word to others, and build the wave of natural healing and preventive medicine. I believe our society would be much healthier and stronger if more and more people practice Qigong and Taiji. Our children would grow up in a more harmonious and peaceful environment. Our seniors would be less dependent on medication. TV would have less violent programs, and more on positive information. I encourage all of you to start Qigong practice today for your own good fortune and good health.

Aihan Kuhn, CMD
President of TQHI

PART I

Qigong and Its Benefits

What is Qigong?

DEFINITIONS

The word *Qigong* (金) is made up of two words, Qi (氣) and Gong (水).

The word Qi has many meanings in Chinese.

Qi is gas, air, breath, smell, weather, manner, spirit, vital energy. As you see, none of these qualities are visible, but all are related to the air or oxygen and mental activity. In this book, Qi refers to vital energy as related to human health and vitality.

Qi, usually translated as energy or vital energy, or life force, is the energy that underlies everything in the universe. In the Chinese character for Qi (氣), we can see the character for rice (土) lies under the character for air (火). When it comes to human energy, there would be no Qi without either rice or air (food and air).

Everything on the earth involves energy. Everything we do involves energy. Without energy, there would be no life. Energy was present billions of years ago, even before the time of dinosaurs. In wartime and other difficult eras, there were many sick people with many problems. As human energy became stronger, society and the economy were also becoming stronger. With good Qi or balanced Qi, you feel healthy mentally and physically. You feel good and have a lot of energy. You feel balanced, less sick, and more productive. There is more joy in life. Good Qi helps everything go more smoothly. With poor Qi, or stagnated Qi, you do not feel well. You feel tired, headachy, stressed out, and depressed. You experience pain and aches; you are always becoming sick; you feel sad or angry. You feel out of balance, not really enjoying life. The symptoms can be both mental and physical.

Qi in every living thing affects everyday life and movement. When we eat food, we need energy to digest and absorb it. It makes sense that you will lose your appetite when your energy is poor or if you are sick. When we walk, do daily activities, or work, we need energy for moving physically and mentally.

Qi refers to the various types of bioenergetic forces associated with human health and vitality. Qi is associated with the lung through breathing, which extracts external energy from air and blends it in the bloodstream with the internal energy extracted by digestion from food and water. The resulting blend is the basis for human energy, metabolism, and immune function. Qi is present internally and externally and controls the function of all parts of the body.

The word *Gong* translates as practice, workout, skill, achievement, and merit. So Qigong conveys the meaning of energy practice, energy workout, or practice to gain skill. The use of Qigong to improve and maintain health was first mentioned in *The Yellow Emperor's Classic of Internal Medicine* written about 200 B.C. The word Gong means not just a simple workout, but also a dedicated workout. You have the same root word in Gong Fu (Kung Fu). It is similar in that it requires a long-term and disciplined workout. When you practice your Gong for a long time, you start to feel the Qi. Qi can be enhanced from practicing Gong. That is why we call it Qigong. You cannot achieve Gong in several days, weeks, or months. If you want to enhance your Qi, you must work hard regularly with your Gong. If you practice a longer time of the Gong, your Qi will last longer and be stronger. Qigong requires a long time or a lifetime of practice before you experience the "true energy science."

Qigong is a traditional energy exercise practiced for many centuries by the Chinese for health, healing, recovery from injury, and disease prevention.

Qi cannot be seen, but it can be felt. Qi involves both the mind and the body. Good mental energy enhances physical energy. If you have poor mental energy with good physical energy, you will soon be falling apart physically; you will have many problems later. Your mental energy has to be balanced first. That is why in China, many cancer patients are healed naturally by doing Qigong exercise. Qigong exercise enhances both mental energy and physical energy, and so contributes to strengthening the immune system to promote healing.

QI AND POSITIVE ATTITUDE

Do you have a good feeling when you talk to a pleasant person who has a positive attitude and good energy? Do you feel drained when you must deal with a person who has a negative attitude and poor mental energy? I do. In my practice, I have seen some people who were very negative about everything; their mental energy was very poor. These people are not likely to improve if they do not try to be more positive. Most people who are very positive heal or improve much more quickly. The best part is they feel much happier. I have seen many students and patients become much more positive after coming to our healing center and taking Taiji or Qigong classes. They enjoy life and cherish life more after studying Qigong and Taiji. Many of my students and patients have become my good friends. Some of them call my center a happy place. By creating strong positive, healing energy in my center, I have been able to witness many people laughing, joking, being more relaxed, and enjoying their lives more. It is really a pleasure for me to see the difference when people begin to make the most of their own positive energy. I think the positive environment at my center helps to bring out the best in people.

I always try to change a person's negative energy to positive energy. In most cases, it works, but sometimes it does not. If I cannot change this person's energy, I have to let this person go to choose their own path, because it not only affects my energy, but also affects other people too. That does not mean I do not want to help this person. There is a saying that "You can lead a horse to the water but cannot make it drink." I do my best to keep my clinic clean and positive so that everyone will enjoy their time there. I always tell people that as long as you want to be better, you have to put your mind to it. Life can always be better.

Several years ago, I had a friend who suffered from depression for many years and took many medications. I tried to help him to find his healing path, but finally I had to give up. His worst problem was being negative in everything and unwilling to change. His Qi was so poor that it affected his life all the time. He had physical problems from head to toe. Since he was not willing to change, no matter how much I tried to help him, I decided to let go of the friendship. It was depleting my energy.

Healing comes from the inside. It comes from your own mind and effort. If you just rely on other people, and not on yourself, the healing does not work and will never work. If you really want to get better, you will find a way to get better. If you only want to complain without trying to heal yourself, the healing will not happen. In Chinese medical theory, if you have poor mental energy, it will block the energy flow in the body and cause both mental and physical problems. People like this are also prone to cancer. On the other hand, cancer patients who maintain good mental energy will live longer and be able to fight the cancer more effectively. If you start working to improve your Qi, you will improve your attitude towards everything and this will bring you more positive energy and happiness.

VARIOUS ENERGY (QI) IN YOUR BODY

Human energy is like an energy network, just like a power station and the power lines that go to different facilities. Human energy includes primary Qi, ancestral Qi, digestive Qi, defensive Qi, internal organ Qi, and mental Qi.

Primary Energy (Yuan Qi): We are all born with primary Qi. It originates from the kidneys and includes kidney Yang and kidney Yin. It is the motor of all organ function. It flows through the meridian system. When a baby is born, the first cry is a sign of this energy. As the baby grows, the energy becomes stronger every year. Sometime we say, "I wish I had energy like that child." You say that because you observe that the child has high energy and never seems to get tired. As the child becomes an adult, he or she starts to deal with more and more stress in life. The Yan Qi must be nurtured with good diet, self care, and coping with stress. For example, he or she does not know how to deal with these stresses, his energy will decline. He will feel tired easily and eventually become sick. If this person knows how to deal with stress, he will be able to maintain his energy. As he continues to grow to age fifty and beyond, his energy starts to dwindle if he does not maintain his Yuan Qi. If this person practices Taiji or Qigong and other exercise on a regular basis, his energy will remain high even after fifty. Just as you maintain your car, your car will last longer and run smoothly, and have fewer problems. This is also true with your body. The human body and mind also need maintenance work. As we become older, our primary energy is reduced faster; that is why we need to pay more attention to self-care. We can use TCM for a tune up and balance treatment. Regular exercise, a healthy diet, appropriate rest, and participating in healthy activities are all important things to help slow down the aging process.

Ancestral Energy (Zhong Qi): This energy is related to lung energy and comes from breathing. A baby before birth has no Zhong Qi. At birth with the first cry, the baby gets first its Zhong Qi in a very weak form, but it becomes stronger as the baby grows. Zhong Qi resides in the respiratory tract and controls breathing. Its health is reflected in the strength of respiration and in the voice. In Qigong practice, it is the Zhong Qi that improves first, and then other improvements follow. If you have poor lung function or poor lung energy, it is a sign of the weakness of your Zhong Qi. Zhong Qi is highly active in human growth and development, as well as in physiologic activity and metabolism. These all are manifestations of the action of Qi. Zhong Qi also has a warming, transforming, containment function.

Efficient Zhong Qi helps singing. Singers need to have good Zhong Qi. If a singer is sick or gets a cold, she or he will not sing well because her (or his) Zhong Qi is reduced from the cold.

Defensive Energy (Wei Qi): It is also called Protective Energy or Guardian Energy, which you receive after birth. Wei Qi flows on the surface of the body and protects you from various diseases. It can be compared to the immune system in Western thinking. When a child is born, he or she has very limited immune function, which has passed from the mother. If we feed this baby with mother's milk, he or she tends to build stronger defensive energy. The mother's milk will give the child stronger Wei Qi than other milk. It is quite difficult to understand the difference between the Eastern and Western theory on this point. It has taken me almost a lifetime to understand these differences, so do not expect to be able to analyze the difference between Eastern and Western theory early in your study.

Children become sick more often than adults because they have lower defensive energy than adults. As a child grows older, he or she develops stronger defensive energy that will protect him or her from sickness. This defensive energy can be strengthened by various exercises including Taiji and Qigong, as well as other Western exercises. Many things such as childhood stress, poor diet or over-eating, no physical exercise, excessive homework, or poor parental support can also weaken this energy. If a child has poor primary energy, he or she will be likely to have poor defensive energy too. Unless he or she really pays attention to build up his or her defensive energy by doing things right to balance life such as, regular exercise, good diet and good parental support, the energy will continue to decline. Taiji and Qigong are very good for building up strong defensive energy.

Digestive Energy (Shui Gu Qi): It is called nourishing energy, which you have at birth. In Chinese, it is also called water and grain Qi. It flows through the meridian system in the body and is related to spleen and stomach energy. It is one of the most important organ energies and plays an important role throughout life. When a baby is born, its digestive system is weak; that is why we feed baby food rather than adult food. As the baby grows, his digestive energy becomes stronger. If his primary energy is poor from birth, he tends to have poor digestive energy too. In Chinese theory, the digestive energy is very important and should not be ignored. In the United States, many people do not pay attention to protecting digestive energy in childhood or adulthood, or both. Overeating is a big problem, and this trend seems to be increasing. The average person eats 50% more than what they should. Many people have indigestion, Irritable Bowel Syndrome, and other intestinal illnesses. The rate of colon cancer and breast cancer is higher in the U.S. than in China. Some people eat the wrong foods all the time. If we would pay more attention to our digestive system, our health condition would be much better.

Digestive energy is fundamental to other energy too. If you have really poor digestive energy, you feel tired all the time no matter how well you eat, no matter how hard you try to become healthy. Sooner or later, your other energies, such as Yuan Qi, Zhong Qi, Wei Qi will diminish. In this case, a TCM doctor or practitioner can help you correct the problem. You can also strengthen the digestive energy by practicing Qigong exercise and self-massage in mild cases. The exercise might not work if the digestive energy has been off-balance for a long time, or in a severe case. You need to take care of this problem by undergoing acupuncture treatments and Chinese herbal medicine, as well as changing your diet.

Improving digestive energy is not meant solely to boost appetite. It is also meant to bring about a balanced appetite, and optimum digestion, absorption, and metabolism. Most Qigong masters have very good digestive energy; they seldom overeat. They have enough energy from practicing Qigong for daily tasks and activity so they do not need extra food for energy. Qigong masters are also not overweight because they know how to keep balance in their life and avoid excess.

Internal Organ Energy (Zang Fu Qi): We have it once the organs are formed even before birth, but it is weak. It becomes stronger as we grow. Each organ has different energy that plays a different role in the body. Though the names are the same, these are not exactly the same as the organs in Western anatomy. For instance, heart energy is related to our mind and spirit besides being directly related to the pumping blood. In Western anatomy, the liver is the place where chemical production, reaction, and breakdown occur. In Chinese medicine, the liver is thought of as storing the blood and is related to mood. All organ energy is interrelated. If one organ has a problem, it eventually affects other organs, just like dominos. That is why we need to anticipate small problems to avoid larger problems later.

Mental Energy (Xinling Qi): The modern definition identifies the relationship between body and mind. The Chinese have been using positive mental energy to overcome many problems for thousands of years. Positive mental energy is essential to our well-being. This is in some way related to the functioning of our organ energy. It is closely related to heart energy and liver energy. In Western terms, we speak of a biochemical imbalance in the body and brain. Xinling Qi is greatly affected by how you were nurtured, your education and continuing education, your social skills (or your EQ), and the values you learned from your parents. It has a significant effect on our immune systems.

Good Mental Energy is very important in our lives, especially our spiritual lives. In the United States, early childhood education is not as strong as in China. This is part of the reason we have so many problems. Children become spoiled. They can have everything they want, or they oppose the parent who does not give it to them without clear and well-defined explanation. When these children grow up, they tend to follow the same path as their parents. They behave the same way as their parents did with them. If we do not pay attention to the parent's education, this will continue generation after generation and will never improve.

Compared to the U.S., as far as I know, the problems of children are much less frequent in China. I rarely hear of children smoking, using drugs or alcohol. There is no teenage pregnancy, and they rarely have violence in schools. Most children focus on their studies, even though they have far fewer material goods than we do here. Most children obey adults and respect adults, especially seniors. Maybe they have other issues that I do not know; I only go to China once a year.

The divorce rate in the U.S. is much higher. Violent crime is much more common here than in China. Depression is much more prevalent, as are problems with teenagers, drug and alcohol addictions, and levels of stress. Part of the reason is the system in this country is incomplete; other reasons come from us. Many people complain about others and do not try to improve themselves. Lawsuits are common even over very small matters. It is always someone else's fault no matter what happens. The law sometimes does not speak for truth and righteousness. Obviously we cannot change the system overnight, but we can change ourselves by working hard on building inner peace and letting go of the negative energy. This way, we can gradual build good and healthy mental energy. We can start to teach our children to do the right thing, to think more positively, to respect others, to help out rather than just take. We can improve our health by doing the right exercise and eating the right foods and by participating in the right activities. We can improve our mental and spiritual health by learning Daoist philosophy, changing our way of seeing things, doing things and dealing with situations differently. How might things be in our society if we always tried to correct ourselves?

I hardly ever saw people suffering from mental illness when I was practicing medicine in China. Here, I see these cases quite often. One of my students was divorced. The divorce was not his choice at first. His wife had many mental problems holding her back; she was never able to move on. She was negative with everything. She would become very upset even in a normal conversation. She never believed in Chinese medicine, Taiji, or Qigong. Since her mental energy was so poor, she also had many physical problems too. The body cannot be separated from the mind. Taiji and Qigong can improve mental energy as well as physical energy. It is an excellent exercise for all ages.

These different energies, work together like the parts needed to build a house. Generally speaking, the Yuan Qi is like the foundation of the house; the Wei Qi is like the bricks; the Zhong Qi is like the pillars; the Shui Gu Qi is like the screws that hold everything together; the Organ Qi is like each appliance; the Mental Qi is like the people who know how to take good care of the house. Therefore, all of the above are important. It cannot be right without any one of them, or if any one of them is weak.

WHAT AFFECTS ENERGY (QI) IN OUR BODIES?

I created the energy circle to explain the factors that can enrich or deplete our Qi. If we follow the positive circle, we will be healthy and happy with very few problems; otherwise, we will have more problems.

Poor diet. A poor diet or overeating can block our Qi circulation. Just think about how you feel after eating a big meal at dinnertime. How did you feel after Thanksgiving dinner? Did you feel tired? Overeating causes a blockage of stomach Qi that affects lung Qi, and spleen Qi. Eventually it affects all of the other organs' Qi as well. That is why

What Affects Energy (Qi) in Our Body?

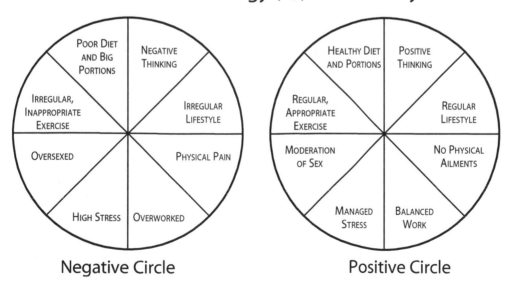

Negative Circle

Positive Circle

some people tell me that they eat too much and never feel well. Eating the wrong food can also cause blockages of stomach Qi. Too much fried food, raw food, or too much meat and dairy will cause problems. It takes so much energy to digest these foods that it exhausts or depletes our stomach Qi. If you eat small portions, it takes much less energy to digest and so preserves your energy for other functions or activity. Many Western scientists do not believe this theory, but they cannot deny the fact that people do feel better and healthier if they follow the healthy Chinese diet and eat small portions. Many centenarians in China have proved this from generation to generation.

Irregular and inappropriate exercise. Many people tell me that they do exercise regularly, but still have physical problems and high stress. Regular exercise is important. The appropriateness of the exercise is even more important. If you only work out with one type of exercise, you gain incomplete benefits; only certain parts of the body get a good workout. If you have a diversified exercise regime such as found in Eastern exercise, you will obtain more complete benefits because Eastern exercise works on different parts of the body. If you have a certain weakness in your body, you need to know what the appropriate exercise is for you. People come to our clinic for many different reasons; we guide them to the right exercise. If you have high stress and anxiety, or high blood pressure, insomnia, headache, Type A personality, I suggest you try Taiji, or Meridian Qigong. If you have physical pain or muscle aches, arthritis, low energy, chronic back pain, stiffness, stomach problems, I suggest that you try Therapeutic Qigong. If you have low metabolism, I suggest that you try power walking or aerobic exercise.

No matter what exercise you choose, you need to be consistent. If you exercise for several days, weeks, even months and then stop, the work you have done will be wasted, and almost all of the benefits you have gained will be lost. You need to continue exercising regularly so that you will maintain these benefits. Western exercise such as walking, jogging, weight lifting, and aerobic exercise can speed up the metabolism, increase the heart rate and blood circulation, and improve muscle tone and muscle strength. They are all beneficial to human health. Eastern exercises such as Taiji, Qigong, and others can reduce stress; improve energy and blood circulation; balance body chemicals; improve balance and immune function; improve muscle resilience, muscle tone, and muscle flexibility; and improve digestive function, breathing, metabolism, and mental focus. Eastern exercises focus on internal energy that gives us the internal strength that will help us in our daily lives. Exercises like Taiji and Qigong bring harmony into our lives and help to keep us well adjusted and happy. Both styles of exercise are important in our lives. If you do both types of exercise, you will have well-balanced health.

Excessive sex. Chinese medical theory states that excessive sexual activity can impair kidney energy, which is a fundamental energy in our body. Kidney energy in Chinese medicine is related to your brain, bone and bone marrow, teeth, hair, and hearing; the kidney stores the essence of the body. Weakened kidney energy affects our daily activity and shorten our life span. Certain signs indicate a weakness of kidney energy, such as low energy, memory loss, appearance of gray hair at an earlier age, arthritis, hearing loss, bone spurs, and low immune function. Chinese Qigong masters work hard to protect kidney energy in their lifetime, especially as they become older. Ancient Chinese health wisdom suggests when you are in your twenties, sex two times a week is all right. When you are in your thirties, sex once a week is wise. When you are in your forties, once in 10 to 14 days is ideal. When you reach your fifties, once in 3 weeks is best. In your sixties, once in 4 weeks is advisable. These recommendations apply especially to men, but are also applicable to women. One can never be a master if one cannot control his or her sexual desires.

High stress. High stress can block liver energy and heart energy that can cause many problems, both physical and mental. In the United States, about 90% of doctors' office visits are for diseases related to stress. Stress weakens our immune function and causes indigestion, Irritable Bowel Disease, insomnia, low energy, poor mental focus, poor daily performance, hypertension, heart disease, anxiety, cancer, and many other ailments. To reduce stress, you should start practicing Qigong or Taiji to harmonize your energy. This harmonization will surely help you to cope with stress. China has a long history of knowing how to deal with stress because the long history of warfare made people work hard in search of inner peace. Practicing Dao gives you an excellent tool for stress reduction. In many cases, stress is caused by imbalanced mental activity and negative thinking, which will be discussed in more detail later.

Overwork. Just think about what happens if you overuse your car. If you drive a car over 200 miles per day, every day, how long will your car last? Our body is not a car, but it shares some of the same principles of maintenance. The human body should be more important than a car. Appropriate work and rest will rejuvenate vital energy so you will be more productive and more focused. Your energy will last longer. Overwork can deplete energy. Not working at all can cause a stagnation of energy. Therefore, a balance of work and rest is very important to maintain human health and a balanced lifestyle.

Physical pain or illness. Any kind of pain or illness will drain your energy and make you both mentally and physically exhausted. Pain is a sign of an abnormality in a certain part of your body. When you have pain in the body, you need to find out the cause of the pain and then work on the cause, not just take medication to reduce the pain. Medication can relieve the pain but cannot help to solve the real problems. Acupuncture is a very good therapy for pain reduction as well as for promoting healing in the area of the pain. Some Qigong can also reduce pain by stimulating Qi and blood circulation.

The illness or pain exhausts your energy and makes you tired; poor energy can cause illness and pain due to the Qi stagnation. In either case, you need to pay attention to correcting the situation before the illness and pain become worse.

Irregular lifestyle. Our body has a natural timer. The 24 hours in a daily cycle have different periods of light and dark and different energy levels. Our body knows when it is time to go to bed and when it is time to start work. Our body's timer follows nature's timer. If we follow our natural timer, our body will maintain a good energy level and function well. If we live opposed to our natural timer, we will lose some of the natural energy. That is why we feel tired if we do not get regular sleep. We need to go to bed at a certain time, not just go to bed at all different times. In China, many people keep the tradition of a mid-day nap. You do not often hear people saying, "I am very tired." Part of the reason is that they have a balanced life with the right amount of resting and working.

A patient came to me asking for help. He had an odd schedule and he was getting only three or four hours of sleep everyday. I told him that he would not get better unless he changed or improved his schedule. In the beginning, he did not believe me; later he was convinced.

Negative thinking. Negative thinking creates negative mental energy that causes your body to drain down and makes you feel unhappy or depressed all the time. Not only does negative mental energy make you miserable and unhappy, but it also makes people surrounding you uncomfortable and difficult to deal with. Left untreated, negative thinking can affect an individual's entire life, leading to a loss of social position, introversion, divorce, and a general lack of enjoyment in life. Negative thinking is harmful to human health and can lead to heart disease, ulcers, muscle pain, depression, violence, and the attendant loss of self-esteem. It can be a source for cancer to grow.

One of my patients who died from cancer was a nice person, but too negative. She was still fighting with her daughter on the last three or four weeks before she passed away. Her liver stagnation was so severe that I could not help her. It was too late. The lesson we learn from this case is that the results would be better if we corrected the problem at early stage.

Practicing Taiji and Qigong can improve energy flow in the body. We begin to eliminate stagnation of energy by increasing positive energy flow. As a person's well-being is improved, he or she begins to feel better. That person begins to develop a positive attitude and to convey that positive energy to others.

Let us look at some ways to resist negative thinking:

Negative Thoughts	Positive Thoughts
"I do not feel well today, I do not want to go out, I do not want to do anything."	"I do not feel well today, but I will continue to do my best. I will be better tomorrow; nothing will get me down."
"She is a nasty person; I hate her. I do not want to talk to her."	"She is not in a good mood today; she might have too much going on in her life, or she may be sick. Maybe she will be better tomorrow. Maybe she needs some help."
"Mary hurt my feelings. I am not going to be her friend anymore."	"Mary hurt my feelings, but I do not think she did this intentionally. Maybe it was just a misunderstanding."

"IT IS SNOWING NOW, I DO NOT WANT TO GO OUT, I CANNOT DO ANYTHING."	"IT IS SNOWING NOW. LOOK HOW PRETTY IT IS! I AM GOING OUT TO ENJOY THE SNOW AND FRESH AIR AS WELL AS SOME EXERCISE SHOVELING THE SNOW."
"HE IS NOT A GOOD TEACHER; I DO NOT WANT TO LEARN FROM HIM."	"HE IS NOT A VERY SKILLED TEACHER, BUT I WILL TRY TO LEARN AS MUCH AS I CAN FROM HIM, HE HAS SOME GOOD POINTS FOR ME TO LEARN."
"I FAILED ON THIS PROJECT; I AM NOT GOING TO DO THIS ANY MORE."	"I FAILED ON THIS PROJECT. LET ME THINK WHAT CAUSED THIS FAILURE SO THAT I CAN IMPROVE NEXT TIME. I HAVE LEARNED A LOT FROM THIS."

One of my patients came to me suffering with depression. She had seen a therapist for many years but was still depressed. Among the many things that were wrong, one that bothered her particularly was that people seemed unfriendly to her. For example, when she was shopping in the supermarket, the cashier gave her a cold look. When she was walking on the street, people passing by would not smile or say "Hi." She felt as if people did not like her. I explained to her the Daoist philosophy and Yin Yang theory, and told her how we can apply these ideas in our daily lives to relieve stress. She was better after our talk. She then started to practice Daoism and Taiji. Her depression was much improved after several months. When she changed, others changed their attitudes to her. She even found a nice guy (before, she had no confidence about herself).

When someone has no smile or a bitter appearance, even a bad temper, first, it does not mean this person dislikes you or is prejudiced against you. Second, it does not mean this person is a bad person. They might be having a hard day, or they might not be feeling well. Maybe their supervisor just gave them too much work and they could not handle it. Maybe their child or other family member is sick at home, and they cannot arrange to go home to take care of them. Maybe they are having problems with their marriage. Maybe they have financial problems. There are many reasons that could make a person unhappy and cause stress in their lives. Some people are able to cope, while others are unable to do so. Some people can control their mood and emotions while others just bring their stress with them to work or to home. If we just try to understand that we live in a stressful society and that people have all kinds of problems, we would not let things bother us. We would be more tolerant. Life is full of the Yin and Yang. That is why we all have good days and bad days. The universe is full of Yin and Yang, that is why we sometimes have beautiful weather, and other times we have thunderstorms or rainy days. If we understand the Dao, the "way," nature, the journey that is life, the path to peace and happiness, we would not let things bother us, no matter what happens in our lives.

One thing I have learned from being the mother of teenage children is to understand the teenager's life. From this understanding, I have developed a tolerance and patience. I let myself be more open to them and let them be open to me. I then can give them the right suggestions and direction. As a wife, I have to understand my husband, a man, just like every man who is different from a woman. I cannot expect a man to think and work the same way as I do. A man's brain process is different. I should not be upset with him when things are not always going as well as I want. With this understanding, I do not develop negative energy.

Changing your way of thinking from negative to positive can help you to avoid much abnormal activity in your mind and create a harmonious environment in your own peaceful world. The key is to be aware of what is going on in your mind. Is it healthy or unhealthy? Taiji and Qigong can help to increase your self-awareness. I believe that if you put enough effort into keeping your mind positive and not let negative energy affect you, you can live a stress-free life.

MAIN QIGONG CATEGORIES

The many different Qigong forms and styles have developed through the centuries. Some focus on the spiritual; some focus on the spiritual and physical. Certain Qigong categories have been popular in China for many years and are still in practice throughout the world.

There are 5 distinct Qigong traditions: 1) Daoist, 2) Confucianist, 3) Buddhist, 4) Martial Arts, and 5) Medical. Each has its own unique style and purpose for practice. Daoism, Confucianism, and Buddhism can be practiced as either religions or philosophies, but you do not have to join a religion to practice their philosophy. Qigong practice can also be approached this way.

Daoist (Taoist) Qigong practice focuses mainly on enhancing natural energy flow in the body. Human beings and nature are considered to be inseparable; humans are seen to be an integral part of nature. Following nature's path and gaining health benefits from natural sources helps to prevent disease and leads to longevity. With practice, we enhance Qi that also comes from nature. Through nurturing and practicing Qigong, one is able to attain inner purification, union with the Dao , and immortality of the spirit. Practice involves both internal (spiritual) and external (dynamic, physical) exercise. Meditation leads to calming and clarity of the mind, which produces insight into the inseparable relationship between humanity and the universe. The Yin and Yang, which should be balanced, is found in every practice of the Dao. In Qigong practice, the mind and breath are particularly important catalysts for connection and change. Furthermore, cultivating personal and moral character assists all internal practices by providing physical, spiritual, mental, and emotional fields that are calm, relaxed, natural, unfettered and energetically strong and balanced. In this state, individuals can cultivate pure self and return to the Dao, which is the way it is supposed to be. Daoist Qigong was further developed from Daoism and represents over 2000 years of Chinese wisdom. The *Dao De Jing* (*Classic on the Virtue of the Dao*) written by Lao Zi (604 B.C.-531 B.C.) was a Daoist bible for Chinese for many centuries.

Confucianist Qigong focuses on mental practice of its ethics and moral character, virtue, and good manners. Through practice, one obtains moral life, creating harmony in relationships, particularly in family as well as the entire community. Cultivating a kind and gentle nature, good morals, love, perfect virtue, righteous behavior, and respectfulness will create a harmonious community and nation. The developing mental serenity and clarity enables one to naturally and intuitively make the right choices or decisions, as well as showing correct manners. This type of Qigong is thought to lead to improved health.

Buddhist Qigong (which came to China along with the Buddhist religion in the 5th and 6th century A.D.) is also concerned with achieving health and longevity as a basis for further spiritual development and enlightenment.

This Qigong, like Buddhist religion, requires internal focus and sitting meditation to cultivate a healthy and strong mind. The focus and meditation work together to reach enlightenment by cultivating one's personal journey of living moderately, avoiding extremes, avoiding desires that cause turbulence in life, and developing love and compassion for all living things. It is practiced more as a still Qigong.

Martial Arts Qigong was developed after the Buddhist monk Da Mo came to China at the Shaolin Temple from India during the Liang dynasty (502-557 A.D.). After Shaolin monks trained Da Mo's muscle and tendon changing Qigong, they improved in both health and martial fighting skills. Since then, many types of Martial Arts Qigong were created to improve the martial effectiveness.

Martial Arts Qigong is more focused on developing and strengthening internal and external energy that shows the absolute power and strength of the practitioner. However, even with extreme external practice, internal practice is definitely involved. Without internal practice, one would lose the external strength. True Martial Arts Qigong practitioners have good moral character and spirit, their energy is long lasting, and they are well respected by all.

Medical Qigong is a combined Qigong form that includes structured, well-designed physical movements that exercise the whole body. Breath control, slow stretching, and self-massage cultivate the internal Qi and blood circulation in organs and other body parts to improve health and eliminate illness. Medical Qigong involves more physical movements. Most Medical Qigong was created by Chinese medical doctors who believe that human health is achieved with a right amount of physical movement, breathing, and self-massage. The Qi station is activated in the body, thereby improving health.

It is Medical Qigong that is beginning to attract a great deal of attention outside of China. Qigong study, which was suppressed during the Cultural Revolution, never died out completely. Today in China, more than 100 million people practice this self-healing exercise daily, especially Medical Qigong. Many people are healed by this ancient healing art. More and more people around the world are becoming interested in this ancient energy practice. Some even go to China to study various Qigong methods and for Qigong healing (hands-on healing). In 1988, the Chinese held the first world conference to highlight Qigong medical research. Since that time, these conferences have grown in popularity and have been held in many other countries. There are many Qigong conferences in the United States each year. Americans are starting to explore the benefits of Qigong practice. In our clinic, Qigong classes sometimes have more attendees than Taiji classes.

All of the above Qigong types share the same basic characteristics:

- Physical or behavioral involvement, mental concentration, and spiritual cultivation.
- Rooted in nature, self-control, simple work with Qi by various methods.
- Deep and slow breathing in every movement.
- Discipline is required in practice.
- Personal development.

TYPES OF QIGONG MOVEMENTS

Regarding Qigong movements, Motion Qigong, Non-motion Qigong, and Half motion half non-motion Qigong are the three main categories of Qigong movement.

Motion Qigong involves non-stop body movements to promote Qi and blood circulation. Some motion Qigong is more difficult than others. You do not have to start with the difficult ones to gain benefits, because some easy Qigong forms also give you many of the same benefits as the difficult ones. You can practice whichever style you like. The Therapeutic Qigong described in this book is a type of motion Qigong.

Non-motion Qigong involves sitting or still meditation to harmonize the body and mind, relieve stress, and create inner peace. Both require specific breathing techniques. Some people do well with still meditation; others cannot sit long because their body becomes stiff. If you have trouble sitting in a position very long, start with half motion Qigong and then move on after a while. This way your body becomes used to it and the sitting becomes easier.

Halfmotion half-non-motion Qigong is in between the other two forms and involves some body movements and some still meditation. Older people often consider this mixture a good one, but not only older people. Everyone can practice this kind of Qigong.

All variations of the Qigong movement forms have great health benefits. We cannot say which one is better. Each person has a different practice experience and preference. Some people prefer motion Qigong, whereas others prefer non-motion Qigong. Many people enjoy the half and half combination. The best way to find out is to try them yourself to find out which type Qigong you prefer.

In my own Qigong practice, I chose motion Qigong to resolve my physical discomfort, half motion half non-motion Qigong for my stress, and non-motion Qigong for my sleeping. This combination works well for me. I also recommend this kind of practice to my patients. I give patients homework, using certain Qigong movements for their specific ailments. For different ailments, I give them different sets of Qigong movements to deal with their problems. Each patient is different, so they need to do different Qigong exercises depending on their illness and needs. People who practice regularly get better results than people who do not spend time practicing at home.

One of my patients suffers from severe allergies; she would pass out from just being exposed to a strong fragrance. She came to me for help after she went to see many physicians who could not help her. I treated her with Chinese medicine and taught her some Qigong exercises that she could also do at home. Several weeks later, her condition had improved tremendously. She is no longer afraid that she is going to have an attack when she goes out. She has only minor symptoms when she is exposed to fragrance. Now she does the Qigong exercises I taught her every day at home.

You might ask me: How can you tell what had helped her, acupuncture or Qigong? In Chinese medicine, the teamwork of doctor and patient is always an important issue. The doctor helps you to get well; you do the right exercise, or eat the right food to support the treatment. This is what maintains the results. If you do things that oppose the treatment, such as inappropriate exercise or eating the wrong foods, your chance of healing is greatly reduced.

Comparing Taiji and Qigong

Many people are aware of Taiji, but not Qigong. Both of them work to improve energy flow, regulate breathing, harmonize body and mind, reduce stress, and prolong life. Both can be used for self-healing and disease prevention. In fact, Taiji is a form of Qigong, a higher level Qigong whose existence most people do not realize. Taiji is more difficult to learn well. Many years of practice are needed before one can become adept. Both of them are excellent exercise for all ages. We should not separate these two. Beginners should start learning and practicing Qigong before learning Taiji. This not a standard rule, you can learn and practice whatever you like. Once you start to feel the Qi from Qigong practice, you will be encouraged to study Taiji. You can start to learn Taiji before Qigong—as long as you already possess patience and discipline.

The following table shows how we can compare these two exercises:

TAIJI	QIGONG
ADVANCED ENERGY WORKOUT.	BEGINNER ENERGY WORK-OUT.
NEEDS FULL CONCENTRATION.	SOME QIGONG REQUIRES A LITTLE LESS THAN FULL CONCENTRATION.
MOVEMENTS, WHICH ARE ARE SLOW AND CIRCULAR, MAY INITIALLY BE DIFFICULT TO LEARN WELL; TAKES A LONG TIME TO LEARN.	MOVEMENTS ARE SIMPLE EASY TO FOLLOW, EASY TO LEARN, AND BECOME REPETITIVE. SOME QIGONG INVOLVES SELF-MASSAGE.
FIVE MAIN STYLES OR FORMS WITH SOME VARIATIONS.	FIVE CATEGORIES, BUT MORE THAN A HUNDRED FORMS.
BREATHING IS SLOW AND DEEP, AND COORDINATED WITH EACH MOVEMENT.	BREATHING CAN BE SLOW OR FAST. IT VARIES IN DIFFERENT FORMS.
IS A MARTIAL ART, BUT ALSO A NATURAL MEDICINE.	IS A NATURAL MEDICINE, AND USED TO ENHANCE MARTIAL ARTS SKILLS.
	CAN BE PRACTICED IN ANY POSITION.
MOST PRACTICE OCCURS IN A WALKING MOTION.	GOOD FOR ALL KINDS OF ILLNESS, NO RESTRICTION.
NOT PRACTICAL FOR SEVERELY ILL PEOPLE.	
BEGINNERS MAY BECOME EASILY FRUSTRATED.	SOME PEOPLE MAY FIND QIGONG TO BE TOO SIMPLE.
SEE RESULTS ONLY AFTER A LONG WHILE.	SEE RESULTS MORE QUICKLY.
IS A TYPE OF SELF DISCIPLINE.	IS A SELF-THERAPY.
PARTICIPANTS ARE USUALLY YOUNGER PEOPLE, BUT IS AVAILABLE FOR ALL.	PARTICIPANTS CAN BE OLDER, BUT IS FOR ALL.

The above summary comes from my own experience in practicing and teaching certain forms of Taiji and Qigong. Since there are many different forms of Taiji and Qigong, everyone's feeling is different, everyone's experience and practice is different, and every form of Taiji and Qigong produces different results. Therefore, you should keep your mind open when you study Taiji or Qigong.

Let us compare the exercises:

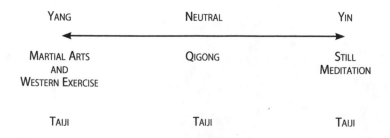

YANG	NEUTRAL	YIN
MARTIAL ARTS AND WESTERN EXERCISE	QIGONG	STILL MEDITATION
TAIJI	TAIJI	TAIJI

Practicing Martial Arts is a Yang-type workout. Meditation is Yin-type workout. Qigong and Taiji are in-between, or neutral. Taiji has all of the above characteristics, Yang, Yin, and Neutral. People can choose from these workout types according to their own needs. Some people prefer sitting meditation, whereas others do not like meditation at all; they prefer Qigong or Taiji. Some people think Taiji is too difficult to learn; others love its challenge. Some people think Qigong is too easy and boring; others think Qigong is the best exercise for them. You must experience each of them before you make a decision about what you want to learn and practice.

Some people have told me that Taiji and Qigong are too slow for them. These people should pay a great deal of attention to their future health because these people seem to be unable to slow down in their lives; They are always on the go and in fight and flight status; they live a fast pace all the time; they do not have balance in their lives. They are prone to heart disease, hypertension, anxiety, and low tolerance in dealing with stress.

Comparing Qigong and Western Exercise

Both Eastern and Western exercise are important in our lives, just like Chinese medicine and Western medicine. We cannot say one is better than the other. They both have an up side and a down side. Both types of exercise can enhance energy, improve circulation, improve immune function, strengthen muscles and tendons, speed up metabolism, reduce weight, and strengthen the heart. If we do both of these exercises, our lives can be more balanced; we will feel so much better. If we just do one type of exercise, our body does not have the balanced strength and energy. Our body and mind gains only partial benefits.

I enjoy both Eastern and Western exercise. I love to hike, power walk, do low impact aerobics, and light weight lifting; but I really enjoy the Eastern exercise more. The latter involves challenges, coordination, mind control, learning, self-discipline, a smooth flow of energy, and the building of a strong life force. Best of all, it helps to reduce stress in our lives and makes us calmer.

Differences between these two exercises:

QIGONG EXERCISE	WESTERN EXERCISE
FOCUS IS ON INTERNAL ENERGY CIRCULATION, CORE STRENGTH, AND MUSCLE FLEXIBILITY.	FOCUS IS ON MUSCULAR STRENGTH.
IMPROVES HEART FUNCTION.	INCREASES HEART RATE.
MOVEMENTS ARE SLOW, GENTLE, AND CIRCULAR.	AEROBIC MOVEMENTS ARE FAST, HEAVY, AND VIGOROUS.
INVOLVES LIFE-LONG COMMITMENT, SERIOUS LEARNING, COORDINATION, AND BALANCE TRAINING.	EASY TO LEARN, MORE REPETITIVE MOVEMENTS, AND LESS COORDINATION INVOLVED. EASY TO DO.
MIND AND BODY WORKOUT.	MORE PHYSICAL WORKOUT.

CONSUMES LESS OXYGEN.	CONSUMES MORE OXYGEN.
EXERCISE INCLUDES BREATH TRAINING.	NORMAL BREATHING BASED ON EXERTION AND TYPE OF EXERCISE.
NATURAL TRANQUILIZER.	NATURAL STIMULANT.
IMPROVES STRESS MANAGEMENT SKILLS.	TEMPORARILY REDUCE STRESS
NO RESTRICTION FOR PRACTICING QIGONG	RESTRICTION WITH SOME AILMENTS
LEADS TO LONGEVITY	NO EVIDENCE SHOWN RELEVANT TO LONGEVITY
QI STAYS THE SAME EVEN WITH AGING.	STRENGTH DECREASES WITH AGING.
PARTICIPANTS: WITH AND WITHOUT HEALTH PROBLEMS, FOR ALL AGES.	PARTICIPANTS: MOSTLY HEALTHY PEOPLE, BUT IT IS FOR ALL.

As we see above, both of these exercise types can be important in our lives.

Qigong Healing and Chinese Medicine

Qigong is closely related to Chinese medicine and is based on the same theories as TCM. Both work on the human energy system to harmonize the body, mind, and emotion. Compared with Chinese medicine, Qigong also works on spirit. Qigong is an integral part of Chinese healing; it is a type of therapy, a disciplined self-therapy that has been used to promote healing for over 4000 years. Qigong is considered to be a natural healing medicine, a preventive medicine, and a longevity medicine. Many people have recovered from long-term illness with diligent Qigong practice. Some consider the results miraculous because they never expected Qigong would help. I had not believed in Qigong before, but now I am teaching and practicing on a regular basis. I have gained many health benefits since I started practicing Qigong regularly.

Qigong is one of the most powerful prescriptions you can receive from a Chinese doctor, because it works directly on the body's energy system. The energy system can boost immune function, balance the hormones and other biochemicals in the body, as well as bring about a happy life. Qigong is a human energy science. In Qigong practice, there is no separation between the body and mind. Just as in Chinese medicine, Qigong helps to heal the mind and the body. If your mind has not been healed, the body will not heal no matter how hard you try. Many things can give us disease, but not everyone becomes ill. Why? We can only refer to this unique human energy science to explain this phenomenon. It is all about Qi. Statistics show that people who do Qigong regularly in China go to the doctor much less often.

Qigong can be used to help relieve or heal many ailments. It is particularly good for healing problems that Western medicine cannot identify. Frequently these ailments involve organ function problems that do not show up on scientific tests. In Western medicine, doctors often look just for abnormal numbers in the blood work or over-grown tissue, or bone on x-ray film or an MRI; but they are less likely to pay attention to the quality of the organs, tissues, and the biochemicals in the body. Normal counts do not mean a person is healthy. Many people who have Qi problems are not healthy even though their test results are normal. The human body is much more complicated than what we know. There is much more for us to explore.

Qigong is very good for correcting immune system disorders. Qigong enhances immune function because it relaxes the mind and the body. In this modern society with its fast pace and stressed life style, our immune system is becoming weaker. Many studies have shown that stress can lower immune function. For these reasons, practicing Qigong on a regular basis means we will be sick less often.

Qigong helps reduce chronic pain and other chronic ailments. In China, medical practitioners in hospitals often prescribe Qigong for treating arthritis, asthma, bowel problems, diabetes, migraine, heart disease, hypertension, high stress, anxiety, and many other disorders.

Once, I had a migraine attack from high stress. The shooting pain was so unbearable that I was nauseated. I decided to practice Meridian Qigong that I also taught in my clinic in the hope it might help my headache. I immediately felt the Meridian Qigong relax an artery in my head. After about 30 minutes of Meridian Qigong practice, my headache and my anxiety went away. I also felt very relaxed afterward.

In China, Qigong has also been used to treat cancer and to reduce the side effects of chemotherapy and radiation therapy. Many people suffering from cancer have extended their lives with Qigong practice or with Qigong therapy. Many patients who experience chemotherapy or radiation therapy feel much better after Qigong practice. Cancer patients gain some hope and light in their lives.

One of my high school friends had lymphoma. The doctor told the family that she might live approximately two to three years. I visited her five years later and she was still in good shape. After ten years, I saw her again. She was surprisingly well. As far as I know, only two things could have saved her life: her persistent Qigong practice and a strong faith.

Qigong practice has been documented to speed recovery from surgery and other kinds of injuries. Many people in China practice Qigong after injury or surgery. They recover faster than those who do not practice Qigong. I used Qigong and Taiji to treat my leg that was injured a few years ago. Now my leg is all better now without having used any medication.

Among all stress management techniques, Qigong and Taiji are the best methods for stress reduction. The reduction happens so subtly, spontaneously, naturally, and with only minimal effort. You just practice Qigong as a daily exercise. You will note that your life changes after a while; your relationship with family and other people improves noticeably; you feel naturally calmer, less irritable, and less anxious. You eventually find out who you are and what you really enjoy in your life. That is why we call Qigong and Taiji natural tranquilizers.

Qigong can be used for healing of any kind of ailment if you do practice diligently. Anyone can do Qigong and find out about its healing power. As we know, Qigong is considered to be a natural healing medicine.

Qigong and the Healing Process

INCREASING OXYGEN IN THE BLOOD AND ORGAN SYSTEMS

When you start to practice Qigong, you start to regulate your breath. Each deep, slow and regulated breath will bring more oxygen to your body, through your lungs to the bloodstream, then to all parts of you body, including the brain, heart, lungs, kidneys, liver, stomach, intestines, spleen, reproductive system, muscle system, glands, etc. The increase in oxygen nourishes and strengthens the organ and enhances the quality or vitality of the organ. Qigong not only increases the oxygen flow in the body, but also improves oxygen usage by organs and tissue. That is why Qigong is considered a natural anti-oxidant that contributes to a delay in the aging process.

HARMONIZING THE CHEMICAL BALANCE

Deep and regulated breathing helps to harmonize the body chemicals including adrenaline, noradrenaline, serotonin, and many other biochemical components. Many illnesses are caused by chemical or hormonal imbalance. Chinese medicine believes that if you use external chemicals to balance the internal chemicals, such as taking a pill to supplement a chemical that is low in the blood, you may actually cause more imbalances by interfering with the body's natural feedback response. Our body has an auto-regulating system, which allows us to be in balance most of the time. If a certain chemical is low, the auto-regulating system will stimulate the corresponding organ to release more of this particular chemical to balance the level. External chemicals suppress this self-regulating system and give false information to the body, so the body stops releasing the chemical itself. That is why a person who takes a thyroid hormone pill will usually have to take it for life, because of the destruction of the self-regulating system of the thyroid gland. If the person starts to practice Qigong consistently or receives acupuncture treatments, he most likely will be able to restore this self-regulating system. Eventually the level of the hormone will be normal without need for ingesting external chemicals.

With Qigong practice, there is definitely a feeling of chemical balance if practice is done right. Qigong involves both motion and stillness. There is stillness in motion; and there is motion in stillness. If Qigong involved just stillness without any motion, it would be difficult for many people to follow. If it were just motion without stillness, we would lose many of the mental benefits of the Qigong and gain fewer benefits than we expect to gain from practice. The deep slow breathing and focus on Qi flow decreases the chemicals that are overly active and increases the chemicals that are underactive.

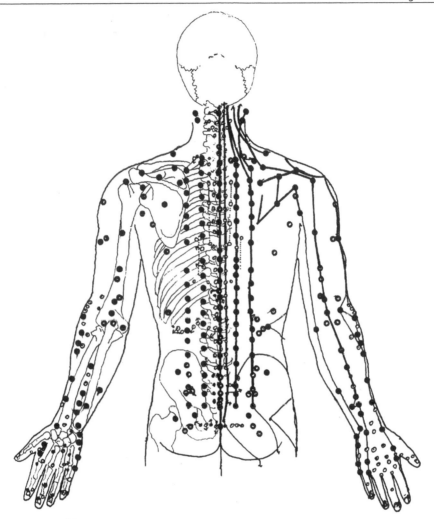

HUMAN MERIDIANS AND ACUPUNCTURE POINTS ARE ENERGY
PATHWAYS THAT CORRELATE TO INTERNAL ORGANS AND ARE USED IN HEALING

That up-and-down is not necessarily just quantitative; it is also a function of the quality of the chemical.

People with hypertension, muscle aches, and anxiety begin to feel improved after practicing Qigong; part of the reason is due to this improved chemical balance.

BALANCED AUTONOMIC NERVOUS SYSTEM

There are two types of nerve systems in the body. The first is the somatic nerve system that makes our body move, feel, think logically, etc. The second is the autonomic nerve system that controls the internal organ system, glands, blood vessels and sensory systems. Qigong not only regulates the somatic nerve system as evidenced by improved mobility of the muscles and joints, but also improves the autonomic nerve system, including sympathetic nerve and parasympathetic nerve system responses. Each deep inhalation stimulates sympathetic system activity, whereas each exhalation stimulates the parasympathetic activity. The more regulating the breath you practice, the more balanced will your autonomic nerve system be. That is why Qigong masters have fewer physical ailments in their lives. They also tend to have excellent digestive systems and immune systems.

OTHER BENEFITS FOR HEALING

Qigong improves the auto-regulating function, in the body's network. Our body parts and organs are like a team. Each part of the body has its own function but also affects other parts of the body. In healthy people, the body regulates itself. For instance, you would eat only when you are hungry and you would rest only when you are tired. Your body would release a biochemical to the blood stream only when this particular biochemical is low in your blood stream. Your body would release certain hormones at a certain time of the month or a certain time of the week; you know how to avoid conflict in certain situations. When you are imbalanced, your auto-regulating system does not work well. You find it is difficult to control your emotions and difficult to stay healthy.

Health Benefits of Qigong Practice

CARDIOVASCULAR SYSTEM

Qi is the motor of the body. Just like your car, the bigger car with the bigger motor will go faster and have more power; the small car will go slower and have less power. The Qi in the body is like the motor. Strong and balanced Qi will maintain good blood circulation with less vascular disease. The rate of heart disease is much lower in China. One of the reasons is that people pay attention to improving the body's Qi circulation. Another reason is they maintain a healthy diet.

RESPIRATORY SYSTEM

Through deep breathing, more oxygen will be delivered into your bloodstream and to your organs. Your respiratory system will receive more oxygen too. The respiratory immunoglobulin called IgA is a type of antibody in your respiratory system that protects you from respiratory infection. Qigong practice increases the IgA in both quantity and quality. In Chinese medical theory, Qigong practice improves the defensive energy described previously. People who practice Qigong are unlikely to get respiratory disease.

GASTROINTESTINAL SYSTEM

When you practice Qigong regularly, the blood circulation improves, more oxygen reaches the organs, and the parasympathetic nerve function improves resulting in your digestive enzymes and other digestive chemicals staying at normal levels. The mobility within the digestive organs mostly stays normal which contributes to natural cleansing.

You will also be able to maintain better digestive energy. Your whole digestion and absorption tends to be normal. You do not need to take extra supplements because digestive energy is balanced. Qigong masters rarely have digestive problems. Many people ask me what kind of supplements I take. They think I have been taking some miracle herbs or supplements. I tell them that I have a hard time remembering to take supplements, but I always do eat healthy foods. I really do not need supplements because I have been following a healthy Chinese diet for many years, including the foods I like and do not like. The most important thing is to practice Qigong and Taiji regularly.

Musculo-Skeletal System

With whole-body continuous movements involving contraction and stretching along with breathing, your muscles get balanced exercise. This is especially true in Therapeutic Qigong. Your muscles receive plenty of oxygen from good blood circulation, and the tissues in your muscular system tend to be healthy. You will have less muscle tension, less degeneration, delayed muscle aging, good muscle resiliency, and flexibility. Healthy muscles and tendons can prevent arthritis, fibromyalgia, and tendonitis. Qigong practice helps to prevent muscle and bone degeneration. Not only will you have fewer pains and aches as well as less stiffness, but also you will have less chance of a fracture occurring when you fall. Your body feels younger even throughout the aging process.

In 1991, I went to China. As usual, I went to a public park in the early morning, where I saw an 82-year-old woman doing Chinese exercise. In the morning practice of her Qigong, she kicked her leg even higher than I could. I then found out she came to this park to do exercise everyday rain or shine. That motivated me to start to work hard with my practice. I thought at that time, if she can do this, so can I. I started practicing hard and started my teaching career in the U.S.

Increased Stamina, Daily Energy Level, and Immune Function

With improved energy flow, your body is at an optimum stage. Your endurance is good and your stamina is strong. A person who practices Qigong is able to work longer hours and still have good productivity. Because of the balanced chemicals in the body, the immune system tends to be balanced too. People who practice Qigong become sick much less frequently. I have seen many students improve their energy level and immune system. They rarely got a cold. Even when they caught a cold, they recovered from it quickly.

Central Nervous System

Because of improved biochemical and neurochemical balance in the body and brain, people who practice Qigong tend to be more focused, respond more quickly to learning, think more logically, maintain mental sharpness and alertness, and improve in their ability to perform daily tasks with great ease. They are less depressed, anxious, stressed, and confused in making decisions. Qigong practice greatly benefits people who have Attention Deficiency Syndrome (ADD). I believe if we start to teach children Taiji or Qigong, they will be able to focus on their academic study and other healthy activities. They will also have healthier mental processes.

OTHER HEALTH BENEFITS

- Qigong practice improves metabolism. You rarely see an overweight Qigong master or practitioner.

- Qigong practice improves balance, which helps to prevent falls.

- Qigong practice not only reduces the risk of cancer, but also assists in cancer healing.

- Qigong practice improves lifestyle and brings more happiness to life.

- Qigong masters are often not stressed out because they know how to avoid negative energy.

There are many other benefits to Qigong practice that are apparent in different people's experiences. I have seen many people in my practice who have had all kinds of good experiences after they began to practice Qigong. Qigong is not magic; all the benefits come from diligent practice and faith, a positive attitude, and patience.

Qigong Research Data

(From QigongDatabase: www.qigonginstitute.org)

Qigong has been used in the treatment of asthma and other ailments. Hua Huang stated in a 1990 paper titled *Clinical Applications of Chinese Qigong Therapy and Its Mechanism*:

> Since 1958, we have used a combination of Chinese Traditional and Western medicine in treatment of chronic bronchial asthma in which Qigong played a primary role. Through four years of short and ten years of long term follow-up, it was found that 99 patients have shown considerable improvements. The effective rate has risen annually. The general effective and the significant effective rates were 93.9% and 69.7% respectively. On the other hand, the 83 cases which stopped their training for six years after persistent training for four years; the general effective and the significant effective rates were only 3.5% and 46.9% respectively. After seeing these statistics it can be said that the results show satisfaction both in short and long terms follow-up. Since 1970, we extended this combined treatment to the following ailments: hypertension, coronary heart diseases, neurasthenia, insomnia, gastrointestinal diseases, pain syndrome, therapy of chronic bronchitis, pulmonary emphysema, and the results are promising also.

Qigong has also been used in the treatment of cancer. In his 1990 presentation at the 1st International Congress of Qigong at the University of Berkeley titled *Prevention and Recovery from Cancer Through the Practice of Guo Lin's "New Qigong Therapy"* Chungsiu Wong stated:

After 20 years of medical experience with qigong, it has been proven that Guo Lin New Qigong is of great benefit for most cancer patients, irrespective of the stages of their illnesses, be it cancer of the lung, breast, throat, stomach, uterus, digestive tract/intestines, esophagus, leukemia or the lymph gland.

Guo Lin's New Qigong is in agreement with both Western and Chinese medical theories pertaining to the treatment of cancer, namely, increasing the ability of the body to resist cancer, restricting its growth, increasing the longevity of the patient and finally eradicating the cancer cells completely.

Through laboratory experiments in China, it has been known that oxygen is the enemy of cancer cells; they cannot exist among oxygen. Guo Lin Qigong therapy increases the oxygen content in the blood many fold.

Results of Patients Treated in the USA with Guo Lin New Qigong

Cancer Type	Number of Patients	Favorable Results(%)	No Results(%)
Lung	23	73.2	26.8
Breast	12	82.2	17.6
Nose	14	61.8	34.2
Intestinal	23	65.8	34.2
Uterine	26	70.5	29.5
Leukemia	43	60.8	39.2

Cancer patient practitioners of Guo Lin New Qigong therapy have experienced optimism, gradual to complete elimination of side effects from chemotherapy and radiation treatments, shrinkage to complete reduction of tumors and even other ailments or chronic disease in the body have been eliminated.

In their 1990 paper *Qigong for Increasing Learning Ability*, Sufang Tong and Peiqi Xe discuss more beneficial effects of Qigong:

Chinese Qigong meditation and physical exercise are well known to improve health and well-being, but Qigong is also believed to improve concentration of the mind and enhance mental acuity and memory. To test the effects of Qigong on learning, a research study was carried out over a period of one year between 1986 and 1987 at an elementary school in Beijing. A total of 170 fourth grade students with about equal number of boys and girls were divided into four groups. For the first 6 months, none of the groups practiced Qigong. During the second 6 months, two groups practiced Qigong meditation, and the other two groups did not. The qigong consisted of sitting meditation for 2 minutes before each class during the day. The students were instructed how to breathe (with their abdomen in gradual, deep, long, thin, even and stable breaths) and to keep an empty and calm mind. During class periods, these students continued to practice this form of Qigong with their eyes open.

The students were given examinations in three subjects (Chinese language, mathematics, and geography) before and after the second 6-month period. Over this period of time, the average test scores of members of the Qigong groups increased from 83.1 to 93.01, corresponding to an 11.9% increase (P-value <0.01). During the same period, the average test scores of members of the non-Qigong groups did not change significantly, 81.6 and 82.02, respectively. One 9-year old boy in the Qigong group had a long history of being very disruptive in class, was not able to concentrate, and had poor average test scores (55%). After 6 months of Qigong, his average test scores increased dramatically (93%), he became better behaved, and his memory improved significantly.

The results of the study are consistent with the concept that Qigong mediation promotes a relaxed and calm state for the body and mind. The brain is more rested and its energy consumption is decreased. Under these conditions, the mind is better focused, mental functions are enhanced, and the individual responds more rapidly to stimuli and remembers more vividly.

Senior citizens can also benefit as described in a 1988 paper titled *Influence of Qigong on the Declined Intelligence of the Aged* by Fuli Sun, Sumping Lei, and Yiai Yan. Here is an excerpt:

Because the average life expectancy of human beings has been increasing, the symptom of declined intelligence, which is common among the aged, brings about more and more problems for many families and society. In order to research the role of qigong in preventing and curing the declined [diminished] intelligence of the aged, we did the following research.

Determination of the intelligence aging level. We made use of the microcomputer and the [interaction] between man and computer in our research. Our test included 7 indexes of fluid intelligence: speed of mental arithmetic, digit symbol, choice reaction time, count, visual number span, tracing reaction and recognition of meaningless figures. We found out the mathematical model of the intelligence aging in 506 subjects and a measuring system for the intelligence aging level was established. It found the subject's aging level and mental physiological age. This method is suitable for mental workers 16-75 years old. The measuring accuracy among the subjects of 50-70 years old is higher.

Cross-sectional investigation. We tested two groups, and in each there were 48 subjects. The subjects in Group I were mental workers who had been doing the qigong exercise for some years. The subjects' conditions in Group II were just the same as Group I [without] qigong exercise experience. The test result showed the qigong exercise could obviously improve people's thinking response, limb flexibility, short-term memory and attention quality and it made the average mental physiological ages 1.62 years younger than the actual ones.

Longitudinal observation. Among the 19 retired mental workers sticking to the qigong exercise for 6 months, we found that 3 items among their 7 indexes of fluid intelligence had been improved obviously. The mental physiological age decreased from 66.3 years (before the qigong exercise) to 65.02 years (after the qigong exercise). This result proves that qigong can really delay the intelligence decline of the aged.

Changes of EEG. Through the spectral analysis and multiple stepwise regression techniques, we created the mathematics model of physiological age of the brain based on 58 subjects' characteristics of EEG parameters. We used this model to calculate the physiological age of the brain for 8 subjects who stuck to the qigong exercise. The result showed that the physiological age of the brain were younger than their actual ones.*

Much Qigong research work has been done in China as well as in the United States. All of the research shows various health benefits with no side effect in all age groups, both men and women. In my teaching, I have noticed changes in my students, such as energy improvement, balance improvement, changes toward a more positive attitude, and less sickness. People are generally happier, more focused, have improved learning ability, and their symptoms are reduced.

Positive Aspects of Qigong Practice

INTENT

The most important thing in Qigong practice is your *intent*. Without this intent, you can never reach your goal. Each one of us has a different reason for practicing Qigong. Some people want to learn and practice Qigong to maintain good Qi so that they are able to be more productive. Some just want to stay healthy. Some like to use Qigong for healing their chronic illness. Some want to use Qigong to maintain inner peace and a happy life. All of the above are good reasons to study Qigong. The key is how serious you are in wanting to reach your goal. Do you really think it is important? On the other hand, are you just trying it to see what happens? If you really think the goal of studying Qigong is important, you are beginning to have intent. Once you have this intent, you will spend time to practice. You will be able to let go of the junk thoughts in your mind. You will be able to focus, no matter what is bothering you. You will be able to distinguish what is right and what is wrong in things that are happening in your life. This is considered to be the secret of Qigong practice. Qigong practice requires discipline and patience, confidence, a positive attitude, and diligent practice.

WELLBEING

The first thing the good Qigong practitioner or instructor should have is a sense of good health. You should maintain a healthy life style, a healthy diet, and a healthy attitude to things that surround you. Otherwise, one cannot be a good Qigong instructor without the basic sense of healing.

If your instructor always gets sick, how much faith will you have in Qigong practice? A Qigong teacher should be a healthy example that shows how Qigong can enhance vitality and immunity. People who practice Qigong on a regular basis should not become sick easily because they would have built strong Qi and immune function.

*The above information is from Qigongdatabase, http://www.qigonginstitute.org/Database.html.

Otherwise, we might say they did not study Qigong well.

A good Qigong instructor and practitioner know how to keep their mood even, no matter what the situation. Attaining this ability takes training, learning, and practicing for a long time. It is not easy for many people; we have emotions, feelings, compassion. It takes a very special training to be able to control your emotions. When you gain control, you will find that life is not that hard to deal with because you are able to use your intellect rather than being controlled by your passions.

Addiction means you are out of balance that you cannot control your life, you are controlled by your addiction. You cannot be an instructor or teacher. Nevertheless, you can try to use Qigong to help you to heal the addictions.

DISCIPLINE AND PATIENCE

You should practice on a regular basis, not just several days, weeks, or months, and then stop. Qigong practice is a lifetime commitment, a unique healing path, especially for people who have chronic issues and need to be more involved and diligent about their therapy. Many people look for a quick fix or a quick cure. That is why so many people take medications. It is all right to take medication for a short period if it gives you temporary relief. It is unwise to take medication for longer periods because of the medication's side effects. Medication goes through your stomach and is absorbed through the small intestine, metabolized in the liver, and excreted through the kidney. These organs could be impaired by the medication after long-term use.

Patience is very important in natural healing. There is an old saying: "If you work hard enough, even a stone will bloom."

Many people do not have the patience to practice the same movements repeatedly for a long time. They can learn the movements quickly, but only on the surface. They take some lessons, and then think they have learned everything about Qigong or Taiji. They break off practice, and then move on to the next project. In both Qigong and Taiji practice, you cannot learn thoroughly enough without diligent practice. The superficial body movements are the easy part; the important part is to practice seriously and consistently to feel the Qi, as well as open the gate of Qi circulation. Feeling the Qi and being able to open the Qi gate require many years of practice for even just one form. That is why we do not think Qigong and Taiji are easy exercises.

Qigong can be used for self-healing and for healing others. In order to heal others, one should really practice Qigong for many years to build true Qi before he is able to emit the Qi to others to activate their energy. This special technique results only from years of training and practice. It cannot be achieved by taking a few classes. Most people do not have the patience for long-term training; they like shortcuts. In Qigong healing, there are no shortcuts, only long-term practice and long-term benefits. Shortcuts can give you short-term benefits that do not last very long. Only dedicated people can become good practitioners or become masters in the future.

You must believe in Qigong if you want to use Qigong for health and healing. Just as you believe your doctor can help you. You need to develop good discipline, no matter what happens in your life you should continue your daily or weekly practice. This means you need to avoid any excuse that interferes with or stops you from practicing regularly. Sometimes it can be difficult because we are human, and our lives are affected by so many different things and distractions. Just keep in mind, you are not the same as everyone else, you are special, a special person does things that not everyone can do.

FOCUS AND CONSERVING ENERGY

Many people get distracted by many different things. You should not get bored with the simple movements. Even though some movements look very simple, they are not simple if you do them right. Many people just do the movements without any focus on internal energy. That is why they are easily bored. Even in Taiji practice, you can get bored. People who get bored or distracted easily will not be good practitioners or instructors.

Many people do things that waste their energy. They are distracted by stress or become upset with insignificant matters. They try to take revenge from others in order to gain or win. They forget that are also losing, because they spend so much of their own time and energy. If you can preserve energy and use it only on valuable activity, you will be much more efficient in whatever you do. You should keep your mind clear and clean, pure, empty of junk, and full of wisdom. You will then be able to find your center and peace. When you find it, the peace is everywhere.

I have always liked the story the thirsty man who was looking for water. A farmer told him that the water was available 100 feet under ground. He should then immediately dig for water. If he quit after 50 feet or even 90 feet, he would still be thirsty. If he continued to dig until he saw water, he would not be thirsty anymore. This story reminds you that even though the journey is long, it is a worthwhile effort. My own healing path has taught me the same lesson.

CONFIDENCE

You need to be confident about yourself and Qigong practice. If you make up your mind, you can put this confidence into action and begin deriving enjoyment from your action. You sometimes might slip a little, but soon you will be back on track, as long as your mind is clear. Qigong has been around over 4000 years with great success. You should be confident about yourself, trust yourself, and stay with your own healing path.

GOOD QI AND POSITIVE ATTITUDE

Anything will go wrong if you keep a negative attitude. Qigong practice does not give you any side effects, but does give you energy. Natural healing of illness takes time and effort. When you start to see the results from the practice, you will know it is a worthy journey that gives you a lifetime of benefits. It might take years or months. You might even become bored after a while, but do not forget that your goal is to improve the quality of your life and you have to work hard to reach your goal. When you look for results, you will not see results. If you do not look for results, the results will be there. There is no need to be afraid to study and practice Qigong. Qigong is not a religion, and no one can force you to practice but yourself. It is all voluntary, just like you shop in a store and choose the merchandise you want. Your positive attitude will speed up the healing process.

When you meet your instructor, you can sometimes sense his or her energy. If he or she is relaxed, has a good attitude, is patient, kind, and a loving person, has a balanced personality with practical and realistic opinions, you will know he or she is the right instructor. If the instructor seems stressed out all the time or has many personal issues that interfere with teaching or practice, you will know this is not the right person to teach you Qigong. If the instructor's Qi is blocked, the negative Qi he has might affect you and other people. He cannot teach well.

Good instructors must enjoy teaching others because this will make you want to be a good teacher and make you learn more. If you do not enjoy teaching, you still can be good practitioner by working on yourself.

Good instructors must be tolerant of anything, including all levels of students. If you just want to be a good practitioner, you must also be tolerant of yourself. You have to give yourself many chances to learn it well, to grasp it. Good practitioners should never say, "I cannot do it" when practicing a difficult form in Taiji or Qigong. Instead, you should say, "I can do it, no matter how long it will take."

Qigong students always respect their teacher as well as other students, even other people who do not practice Qigong. Respect is a part of practice. If you do not respect others, how will you gain respect from others? I respect my teacher and my mentor a great deal, I am thankful to them for giving me their knowledge and encouragement.

MODESTY

A good instructor never thinks, "I have learned enough," but always wants to continue to learn more about the fundamentals of Qigong. Many people think that if they take some lessons it is enough to teach others. It is acceptable to teach others with what you know. Everyone is able to teach something at different level. However, the more you know, the better instructor you will be, and the better quality class you can offer. Otherwise, you will find your knowledge is quickly exhausted, and you may not be able to answer people's questions. Especially in healing and health care, people have many questions. If you have a greater knowledge, most times, you will be able to answer any questions your students might have for you, and so you will not be embarrassed. Learning is big part of teaching. Once you are in a teaching position, your learning is endless. You also learn from teaching.

A person who loves people has the quality to be good teacher. Just like a school-teacher, if you love children, you can be a very good teacher because you put your heart into teaching and you want your students to learn. You care about people, you want to help people, and you do not care even if you sometimes have to make sacrifices. This should apply to any kind health care practitioner. If your heart is there, your work will be more effective.

FEELING THE QI

In some cases, you use your commonsense to determine the truth, especially if you have practiced Qigong for a while. You develop a sense for identifying what is real or what is not real Qigong. Sometimes you might make a wrong judgment, but if you try it out for a while you will feel it and make the right judgment. Do not be afraid of trying. There is an old Chinese saying: "If you really want to know the taste of an apple, you must take a bite of the apple." Try it; join a Qigong school or group and practice with them; see if you can feel the Qi. If you do not feel anything, you might be doing it wrong, or it may not be the right type of Qigong for you. In our school, almost every student feels the Qi. Feeling Qi might be a feeling of heat, a force in the air, strength, tingling, or a sudden surge of energy. Each person's perception of it is different. Some people have even said to me, "I am having a hot flash." We then joked that Qigong can cause hot flashes. Normally you will feel very warm in your hands and then in your body, but it is not just sweating as if you just went to the gym. Qi energy is much longer lasting than the energy you feel after working out in a gym.

In the beginning, you might not feel the Qi, but after a while, you might feel heat or tingling, or some kind of strange feeling on your hands or body. You should avoid negative thoughts when you decide to practice Qigong or use Qigong as part of your life. If you become frustrated from not seeing any changes in a short period, you are wasting your time. Low confidence and a negative attitude create negative energy, which will interfere with the healing process. This interference is similar to not following the instruction of your doctor if you do not like the doctor. If you practice without any disturbance or interference, practice without looking for results and have faith, you will feel a big difference after a while. You will then realize that

- Your energy level will be higher.
- You will be able to focus better.
- You will feel less anxious or depressed
- You will feel happier and have better relationships with your family and other people.
- You will have less sickness in your life.
- Your chronic complaints will lessen.

INSTRUCTOR'S KNOWLEDGE AND HONESTY

The knowledge of Qigong, human energy, and energy healing is very important. The more the instructor knows the better quality he or she will have, especially if he or she is able to answer your questions correctly. For instance, suppose you ask the instructor, "What kind of Qigong practice is good for fibromyalgia? What kind of Qigong is good for heart disease? What kind of Qigong is good for my back?" If the instructor is unable to answer the question, he or she has not studied enough to know the various kinds of Qigong. The instructor should understand the principles of TCM and understand how Chinese medicine works because Qigong shares many of the same principles as Chinese medicine. To know the difference between Taiji and Qigong is also important because people ask this question quite often. If the instructor cannot answer your question, he or she should be honest with you and tell you where you can find the answer, or he should research the answer for you.

The instructor, even while teaching, should continue his study of this unique energy science with masters. It is all right to study under different masters as long as the master has a good reputation and is of high quality. Unfortunately, not many instructors are willing to spend the extra time to study hard and become very good at this energy science. Most of them study superficially, just enough to teach others some movements. I have been practicing energy healing for over 20 years, but I still continue my study every year in China under a well-reputed grand master because I know this is a lifetime journey for me. Learning should never stop. I have trained many instructors too; only a few have continued their study.

Both Taiji and Qigong are related Daoist philosophies. Knowledge of these philosophies is very helpful in assisting your study of Taiji and Qigong. It helps you to see things more clearly and understand better. You can also apply these philosophies in your teaching as well to enhance your personal enlightenment. You will be surprised to find out how much you will enjoy it, and how much it make sense with everything in our lives.

Before becoming a good teacher, you must be a good student. If you cannot be a good student, you can never be a good teacher. Being a good student is the base or foundation for becoming a good teacher.

What You Need to Know About Qigong

Qigong is not a religion. Qigong does share some similar aspects with religion. Both involve a belief that some benefit will be achieved as a result of practice. However, Qigong is not intended as a religion. Nevertheless, religion can be said to be a type of Qigong. Qigong is simply a workout to improve your mind, body, emotion, and spirit. Religions involve belief and meditation (prayer) while Qigong involves belief and moving meditation. Both are beneficial to our health if used with the right attitude. Qigong offers much more than just belief and meditation: Workouts have an enormous affect on the body's energy system, bringing beneficial changes to body chemicals and physical strength. Religious people worship God; Qigong people respect and love nature. Religious people believe in good and evil; Qigong people believe everyone is born pure. As we grow, things surrounding us change, and that makes us change too; some change toward the right direction, and others change toward the wrong direction. Qigong practitioners can be religious; religious people can also be Qigong practitioners. There is no restriction between these two. Also very important in Qigong practice is your mental, emotional, and physical health. These should be well balanced to promote smooth Qi flow in your body. People who practice Qigong also do not confuse Qigong and God. We do not say, "God makes us practice." We practice because of our own wants and needs.

Even though some religious groups practice Qigong in their own way, they are still working on themselves and not on other people. Qigong masters and practitioners never try very hard to convince others, but instead suggest or tell others about the health benefits they gain from Qigong practice. Qigong practice is purely a self-healing method for health purposes. People who practice Qigong usually have a better understanding of life, are able to deal with stress, and have fewer physical complaints. They are tolerant, easy going, relaxed, have fewer problems in life, and have fewer material desires and more spiritual desires. They see everything in a positive way. The quality of life of the Qigong practitioner or Qigong master is much higher.

Qigong is not a superstition. There is no superstition involved in Qigong practice. There should be no false belief in Qigong practice. All you believe is that your effort can make a difference. You believe that you can always make it better. Sometimes you do hear people saying that miracles have happened. As you know, anything can happen in life, but there is no guarantee. Seemingly miraculous things might happen on occasion, but not to everybody. Human energy science is relatively new in the West. It is often difficult for some to grasp. That is why most Western scientists will not accept Qigong or Qigong healing. Western culture is used to seeing proof from a scientific point of view. They want to see the results from testing. However, how many Western scientists are truly interested in looking into the study of this mysterious energy science?

I wrote letters to 20 Western doctors asking them if they would be interested in joining our TQHI (Taiji and Qi Gong Healing Institute) for a Qigong study on asthma healing. Only one actually responded. Not one told us they would like to join this study. Why? How many of them are open to natural healing?

No political involvement in Qigong practice. In Qigong practice, there is no political aspect. It does not matter if you are communist or capitalist or apathetic, you can still practice Qigong. The masters do not screen who is who, bad or good, by the color of your skin, what type of religion, or how old you are. As long as you really want to study Qigong and are willing to work hard on your practice without bringing your personal political opinions to class, you will be accepted. If you see anyone trying to combine politics with Qigong practice, he does not belong in the Qigong group. He or she cannot learn Qigong well. We all have different opinions about government and the things that surround us; we can talk about these things outside, but not during Qigong practice. One very important aspect of Qigong practice is to keep your mind open, clear, and pure.

All voluntary and not under pressure. Qigong practice is completely voluntary. No one should force anybody to do Qigong. You are in charge of your own health; no one should interfere in your life. Being under pressure to practice Qigong will never have good results. If you understand Qigong, your practice may be easier. You can start reading some books about Qigong before becoming involved with Qigong.

Qigong was never intended to be a big money maker. In Chinese tradition, the Qigong master will not teach a person who has money but has no intention and discipline for practicing Qigong. Masters want to teach people who have a good moral character and good discipline for practice, even if they are poor. Qigong is meant to promote health, happiness, and longevity. It is supposed to be a healthful public activity. Qigong classes should not be expensive; they should be affordable. Most people learn Qigong from taking the class, and then practice by themselves at home on a regular basis. If you do not have this kind of discipline to practice alone at home, you will need to come to class more often and on a regular basis. Even if you have to come to class more often, it should still be affordable. If you find a Taiji or Qigong school that overcharges, they are not true practitioners or masters because they just use Qigong for making profit. Their teaching of Qigong has a different purpose than healing. In this country, the cost of living is much higher than Asian countries; the fee may be higher but will still be affordable. The instructors should realize that they also benefit from teaching because they are practicing at the same time.

If all you as an instructor can think about is how to use Qigong to make a big profit, that is wrong because you will lose compassion, lose the Qi mind, lose the ability to learn, and lose the ability to share with others. If you have good intentions to learn, you will develop good will, good fortune, and a good reputation. You will have a good following, and the good attendance at your classes will be your money source. First, you need to plant the seeds without want or desire. You will harvest the rewards later after your hard work.

PART II

Therapeutic Qigong

Introduction

Therapeutic Qigong is a form of Medical Qigong that was created in the early 1970s by Dr. Zhuang Yuanmin and other Chinese doctors and professors at the University of Sports Medicine in Shanghai, China to assist healing of various ailments. This therapeutic exercise regime is based on ancient Chinese exercises of Dao Yin, Yang Shen, and Qigong, (such as the Leading the Qi method), and Martial Arts, which involve Qi circulation (Life Force). This form of Medical Qigong combines physical exercise, stretching, breathing, self-massage, and traditional therapy to help relieve illness and prevent disease. By enhancing energy and blood circulation, it accelerates the body's healing process, immunity, and longevity.

The exercise regime is divided into several sections focusing on different parts of the body. It combines deep breathing with whole body movements and stretching to promote energy flow and harmonize the mind and body. One can isolate certain movements according to one's needs. Self-massage is also used to activate the meridian system and to relieve and prevent illness and discomfort. In my 10 years of teaching experience, I have seen many people receive health benefits, both physical and mental, from illness and disease such as heart disease, high blood pressure, arthritis, fibromyalgia, back pain, neck and shoulder problems, stomach problems or indigestion, headache, insomnia, depression, anxiety and much more. Even cancer patients have done very well, and some have remained cancer free for many years.

Clinical Studies in China. Clinical studies have shown the tremendous improvement in patients who have practiced these exercises every day for three months. Patients who suffered from neck, shoulder, back, and leg problems were studied. Group A patients underwent massage and herbal therapy without exercising. Group B patients underwent massage therapy and practiced Therapeutic Qigong exercises at home everyday. Three months later, 10 % of group A patients had a complete recovery, 50% improved, while 25 % of group B patients were in complete recovery and 75% improved.

These results were described by Ming et al. in *Medical Qi Gong and Practical Method Gong Fu* in a 1990 publication from the Shanghai Science and Technology journal. These statistics show that this kind of Qigong has medicinal value; it is used as alternative medicine, or assistant medicine.

Observations in the Chinese Medicine for Health clinic in Holliston, Massachusetts

- Ammi Chen, 68 years old, was diagnosed with angina pectoris. During one year, because of the severity of the angina, emergency room treatment was required 3 times. After practicing Therapeutic Qigong exercises daily for 2 years, she has not had any angina attacks. Her EKG is reported to be normal.

- Kenny Healan, 59 years old, had hypertension (high blood pressure) for 5 years and was under medication. After 3 years practice of Therapeutic Qigong Exercise everyday, his blood pressure has returned to normal without any medication.

- Agnes Hung, 45 years old, had chronic back pain for a long time. She felt exhausted after work everyday. After practice of Therapeutic Qigong Exercise for two years, She is totally free of pain and is full of energy at work.

- Joe Smith, 48 had low white blood cell count for several years. After practicing Therapeutic Qigong for two years, his blood count returned to normal.

Getting the Most Out of Your Qigong Practice

You should be aware of these when you practice; it may be more beneficial if you understand what you should or should not do.

Belief in Qigong. You will not achieve good results if you do not believe in Qigong. Just think when you go to a doctor and you do not believe in this doctor, you will tend not to follow his or her instructions, or perhaps you might not want to go back again. If you do not believe that a vitamin is good for you, you will not even take it. If you do not believe in something, you should not do it because it will not work.

Water. Drink water before your morning practice. In the morning, all of the organs in the body are functioning at a low level. Half a glass of warm water is a mild wake-up call. The water will benefit the stomach function by flushing the old stomach juice. We call it "a little cleansing work."

Uninterrupted practice. Practice should not be interrupted. Once you start practice, you actually start moving the Qi. The moving energy needs a certain amount of time to accumulate. If you are interrupted during practice, some of the Qi that you create will be lost, and you will have to start again, which is a waste of time. You should set up the time for practice, and tell your family or children not to interrupt you.

Relaxation. You should be relaxed, not tight, during practice. Relaxation is the most important issue in Taiji and Qigong practice. If you are tight, anxious, or nervous, you will not be able to create this special Qi, so your practice is somewhat useless. Once you reach full relaxation, you will gain full benefits from the exercise.

Compass directions for individual practice. A female should face south, and a male should face North. (This might be related to the magnetic atmosphere on earth.)

If you do not know where south or north is, you can choose the direction for which you have good feelings. This is called "self-judging the Feng Shui." Sometimes it works even better because it fits in with your energy.

Location. Practice in a natural setting is best: green trees, green lawn, flower gardens, botanic gardens, a water source (better with moving water), or any place in nature that make you feel good. Practicing under a full moon at one time was an amazing experience and helped me to get rid of my anxieties.

Frequency of practice. Three to five times a week is good, but it is best to practice every day. Many Chinese people in Mainland China practice Qigong every morning in the park, year after year, generation after generation.

Regularity in practice. Set up a time and duration: It is important to practice at a regular time. If you have time in the morning, you should do it every morning, not one day in the morning, another day in the afternoon. You should also set up a standard time period, either a half hour or one hour, even 15 minutes, as long as you always do the same length of time.

Air quality. Do not practice if the air in the room is not good: Qigong involves breathing. When the air in the room is not good, it will affect the air in your lungs. Poor air quality interferes with your energy flow, and it might trigger your asthma or headache.

Wind. Avoid heavy wind during outdoor practice, because heavy wind distracts your mind as well as removing energy surrounding your body. Heavy wind takes away the energy that you created; it also causes blockage of energy flow in your body.

Elimination. During practice, it is important not to hold the bowels and urine. Doing so causes blockage of internal organ energy flow and your practice will not work well.

Hunger and Overfullness. Do not practice when you are hungry or overfull. Hunger during practice will deplete your energy. You might experience dizziness, a headache, or feel weak after practice. An overfilled stomach blocks the energy in your body. Your Qi will not go though the channels. Your practice becomes a waste of time.

Sleep. Lack of sleep will affect results. A good night's sleep is important. You should always maintain a good habit of sleep time which helps to maintain balanced energy and gain more power from practice.

Clothing. It is better to wear soft cotton clothes and comfortable shoes. The hard cloth and shoes block meridians on your body and feet, bringing about distraction and less effective practice.

Avoid wearing a hat when you practice. Certain movements involve bending forward and backward. Your falling hat will distract your mind and interfere with your practice.

Colds. It is fine to practice Qigong when you have a light cold. If you have a bad cold or flu, you should just rest. The severe illness depletes the energy; you need to restore the energy from resting and not overburden the body. You will not have good results if you practice Qigong during severe cold or flu.

Alcohol. Do not practice after drinking. Alcohol disturbs the Qi flow. A good Qigong practitioner does not drink too much.

Sex. Avoid too much sex. Too much sex can deplete your kidney energy for both male and female, especially male.

Diet. Eating small portions is best; being a partial or half vegetarian is ideal. The reason to be vegetarian is to preserve digestive energy, which plays an important role in maintaining good health and longevity. Eating too much meat can cause stagnation and other health problems.

Qigong forms. Focus on one form of Qigong before practicing another form. Make sure you can master one type of Qigong before you practice another one. You might become confused or distracted if you try to do too much simultaneously. You then will lose the Qi. If you focus on one form, you can really learn and master this form; you will then start to feel the Qi. This Qi will give incredible health benefits.

There is an old saying: "You get out what you put in."

Ancient Chinese Wisdom says to avoid these when practicing Qigong:

Cigarettes—Qi is in turmoil
Alcohol—Qi flows away
Hot spicy food—Qi disperses
Anger—Qi moves up
Being hurried or anxious—Qi rebels
Being overworked—Qi depletes
Being startled or frightened—Qi falls to bottom
Being worried—Qi becomes tangled

Starting Qigong Practice

Therapeutic Qigong exercises are divided into six groups. Each group focuses on different muscles and joints to achieve maximum benefit.

Group A focuses on the neck and shoulders.
Group B focuses on the back.
Group C focuses on the lower back, hips, and legs.
Group D focuses on arms and legs.
Group E focuses on hands, wrists, and elbows.

You do not have to do movements that you give you trouble. You can focus on the movements that help your problems. Keep in mind, if you do all groups (the whole set of 36 movements), you will be starting to work with your true energy system, accelerating the healing process of the body. This will give you the maximum healing benefit.

To obtain these healing benefits, Therapeutic Qigong exercise should be practiced a minimum of three or four times per week, preferably every day. You should do this kind of Qigong accurately. Some other types of Qigong might not require accuracy of the movements.

Before starting, you should be completely relaxed. Focus on breathing to keep your mind free of troubling thoughts; relax your shoulders, chest, waist, legs, and feet. Your whole body should be relaxed and free of any tension. Breathe slowly and deeply. With each deep inward breath, you are taking in more oxygen. Think positively and feel positive energy flow through your body. With each exhalation, you are letting out carbon dioxide and other gaseous wastes, as well as your worries, tension, anger, stress, illness, and negative energy. You should have the feeling of being warm, safe, comfortable, and at ease. You should leave everything behind and not let anything disturb you or interrupt you. In each movement, you do, you need to stretch as far as you can. Each movement requires correct breathing. The breathing patterns are described more fully in the section, Step-By-Step Instructions.

You only need to take 30 minutes a day to go through this form of Medical Qigong. If you only have 15 minutes, you can do first part, which includes 18 movements, and then do the next 18 movements the next day. You can also do just the movements that relate to your particular physical problems. For instance, if you have more problems in the shoulder and neck areas, you can just focus on Group A movements for 15 minutes. It is recommended that you go through the whole sequence of 36 movements for the maximum healing benefit.

Therapeutic Qigong is easy to learn and easy to practice. There is no need for a special place or equipment for practice. The only thing you need is discipline and persistence, especially those people who have a medical condition.

There is neither age limit nor disease limit. Anyone, regardless of their disease, can benefit from this ancient healing workout. We also offer instructor-training programs for this type of Qigong every year. The instructor training program is meant to help provide quality instructors so that more people can benefit from this beautiful healing art.

The first section consists of three parts. Each part involves six movements. The first part helps to prevent and heal neck, shoulder ailments. The second part helps to prevent and heal upper and lower back problems. The third part helps to prevent and heal hip and leg problems.

The second section consists of three parts. Each part involves six movements. The fourth part helps to prevent and heal joint problems. The fifth part helps to prevent and heal tendonitis and bursitis. The sixth part helps to prevent and heal imbalances of internal organs.

Step-by-Step Instructions

Section I

Group A.
Helps to relieve and prevent neck and shoulder problems (including arthritis, bursitis, stiff neck, frozen shoulder, tendonitis, ligament and other soft tissue degeneration, and cervical spondylosis).

---

1 *Slow neck motion*

1. Place your feet together. (Figure 1-1)

2. Breathe evenly through the body from the Baihui point (on the top center of the head) to the Yongquan point (on the bottom of the feet).

3. Slowly step to the left, and center your weight. The distance between the feet should be shoulder width.

4. Put both hands on waist, shoulders relaxed. (Figure 1-2)

5. Slowly turn head to left and inhale. (Figure 1-3)

6. Return head back to center and exhale.

7. Turn head to right and inhale. (Figure 1-4)

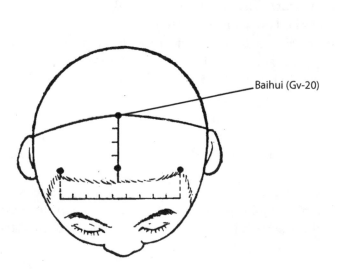

The Baihui (Gv-20) Cavity

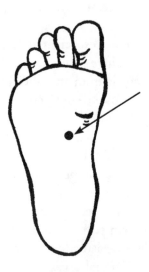

The Yongquan (K-1) Cavity

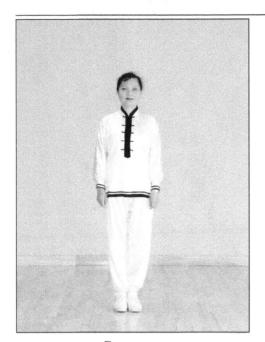

FIGURE 1-1

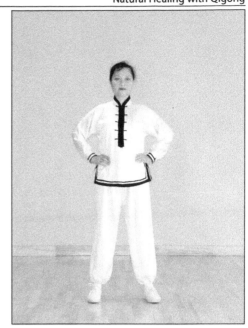

FIGURE 1-2

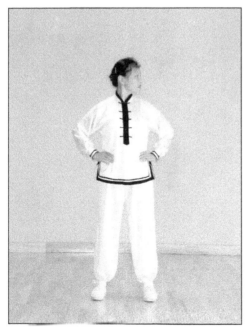

FIGURE 1-3

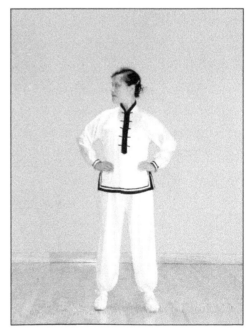

FIGURE 1-4

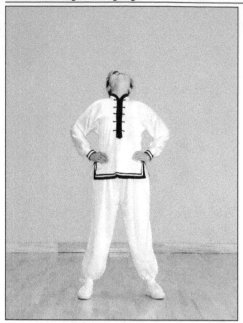

FIGURE 1-5   FIGURE 1-6

8. Turn back to center and exhale.

9. Move head upwards and inhale. (Figure 1-5)

10. Move head back to center and exhale.

11. Move head downward, and inhale. (Figure 1-6)

12. Move head back to center as in Figure 1-2 and exhale.

Important: If you have neck problems, you should repeat this exercise every day for 8 cycles. Stretch as far as you can. Keep your head straight.

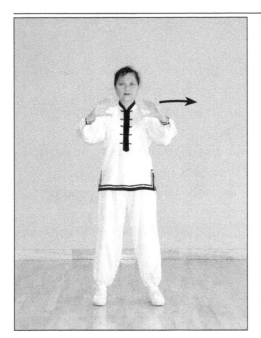

FIGURE 2-1

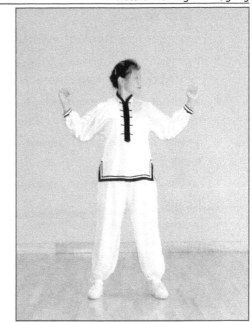

FIGURE 2-2

2 *Horizontal arm stretch*

1. Place your feet shoulder width apart.

2. Lift arms up in front of you with a slightly bent elbow position at chest level. (Figure 2-1)

3. Hold hands in a fist position, stretch arms to the side as far as you can, elbows pointing downward, eyes following to left when stretching arm to side. (Figure 2-2)

4. Bring hands back to front position while exhaling, eyes following back to center.

5. Repeat Steps 1 through 4 except with eyes following to the right when stretching arms to the side. Do this 4 times. (Figure 2-3)

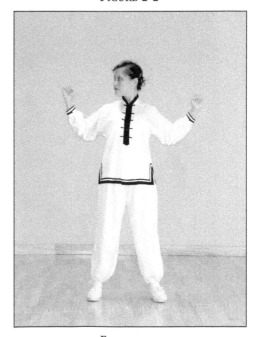

FIGURE 2-3

Important: Remember to stretch arms as wide as possible, and breathe deeply. Inhale as you stretch to side, exhale as you move hands back.

3 *Vertical arm stretch*

1. Place your feet shoulder width apart.

2. Place arms on the side of the body with slightly bent elbows and elbows pointed down, fist up. Shoulders should be relaxed. (Figure 3-1)

3. Breathe in deeply and slowly, slowly raise hands up, palms facing front, eyes following the left hand up. (Figure 3-2)

4. Breathe out and slowly move arms down, eyes following the right hand down.

5. Take a deep breath and raise hands again, eyes following the right hand up. (Figure 3-3)

6. Breathe out and slowly move hands down, eyes following left hand. (Figure 3-4)

7. Repeat above movements.

Important: Raise hands up as high as you can, with arms straight, breathing deeply and slowly. Breathe in as you raise hands, breathe out as you lower hands.

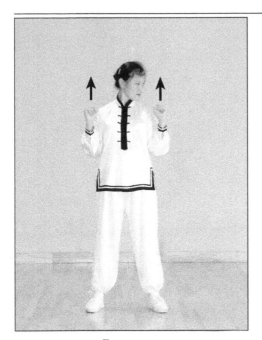

FIGURE 3-1

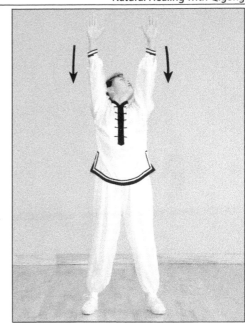

FIGURE 3-2

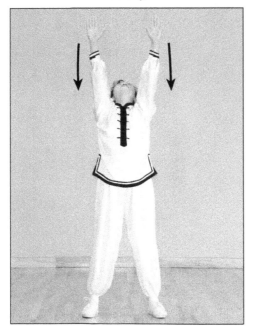

FIGURE 3-3

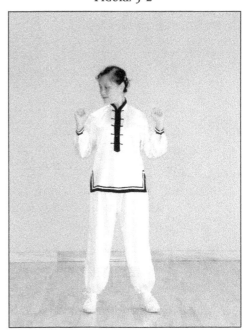

FIGURE 3-4

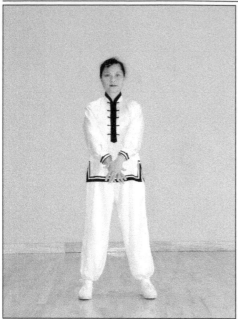

FIGURE 4-1

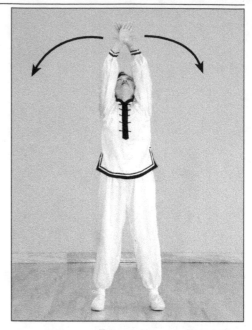

FIGURE 4-2

4 *Rotational arm stretch*

1. Place your feet shoulder width apart.

2. Overlap hands in front of you. (Figure 4-1)

3. With arms straight, slowly raise hands until they are over your head, breathe in deeply, eyes following hands up. (Figure 4-2)

4. Separate hands, let hands fall to the side of your body keeping arms straight, eyes following left side. (Figure 4-3)

5. Again overlap hands in front of you, slowly raise hands up with arms straight, inhale.

6. Separate hands and slowly move hands down to the side, exhale, eyes following right hand.

7. Repeat above movements.

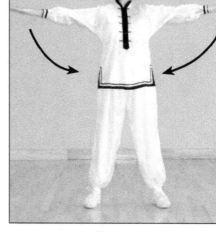

FIGURE 4-3

Important: Straighten and stretch arms as far as you can, as back as you can. Breathe deeply, slowly and smoothly.

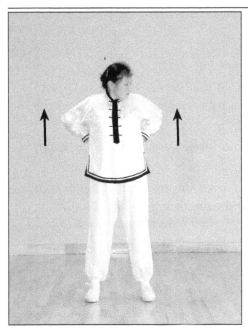

FIGURE 5-1

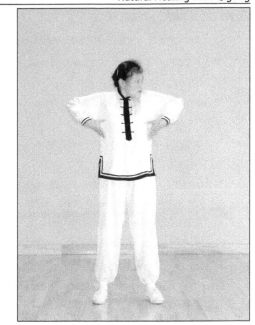

FIGURE 5-2

5 Angel-wings shoulder rotation

1. Place your feet shoulder width apart.

2. Put both hands behind lower back with palms facing inwards but not touching the body. (Figure 5-1)

3. Inhale and slowly raise shoulders and hands along the side of the spine, lifting shoulders as high as you can, eyes following left side. (Figure 5-2)

4. Exhale and slowly move hands to front of the body, relax shoulders and palms press downward. (Figure 5-3)

5. Inhale and slowly raise shoulders and hands along the spine, lifting shoulders as high as you can, eyes following right side. (See Figure 5-1)

6. Exhale and slowly move hands to front of the body, relax shoulders and press palms downward. (Figures 5-2 and 5-3)

7. Repeat above steps.

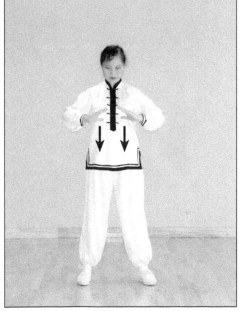

FIGURE 5-3

Important: Breathe in and out deeply and move shoulders to their maximum.

6 Arm and side stretch

1. Place your feet shoulder width apart.

2. Place right hand on lower back with palm facing out.

3. Inhale, slowly raising your left hand up from the left side (Figure 6-1) until it is above the head with arm straight and palm facing up, (eyes follow the left side up). (Figure 6-2)

4. Exhale, slowly move left arm down behind lower back, above right hand, palm facing out.

5. Inhale, slowly raising your right hand up from the right side (Figure 6-3) until above the head with arm straight and palm facing up, (eyes following right hand up). (Figure 6-4)

6. Exhale slowly, move right hand down behind lower back, above left hand.

7. Repeat above movements.

Important: Breathe deeply. Keep your back straight.

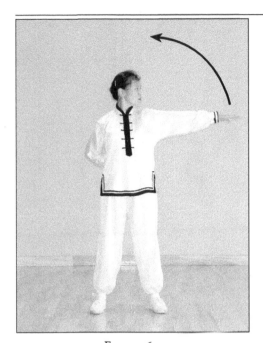

FIGURE 6-1

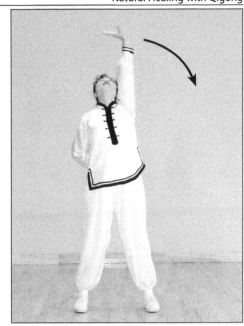

FIGURE 6-2

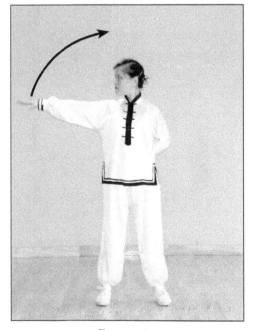

FIGURE 6-3

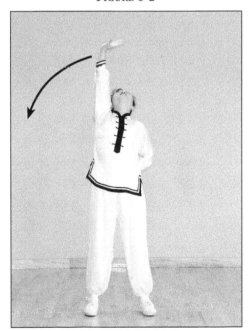

FIGURE 6-4

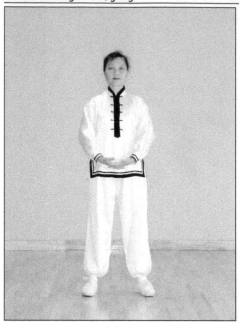

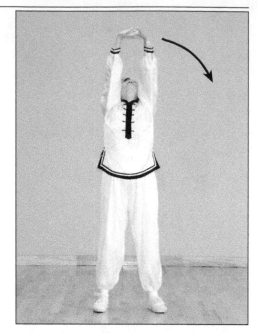

FIGURE 7-1   FIGURE 7-2

Group B.
To prevent and help relieve back problems (including: chronic back injury, contusion, arthritis of spine, soft tissue degeneration, disc problems, and muscle spasms).

7 *Holding sky and side swing*

1. Place your feet shoulder width apart.
2. Interlock fingers in front of body (Figure 7-1), inhale raise hands up above your head, arms straight, palms up. (Figure 7-2)
3. Exhale, slowly bend upper body to the left (Figure 7-3), then up straight.
4. Bend body to left again, then up straight.
5. Exhale, separating hands to your sides (Figure 7-4) and down, eyes following left hand down.
6. Repeat Step 2.
7. Exhale and slowly bend upper body to right (Figure 7-5), then up straight.
8. Bend body to right again, then up straight.
9. Exhale and separate hands to your sides (Figure 7-6) and move hands down, eyes following right hand down.

Important: Keep arms straight when fingers are interlocked above head and keep hips still. Do not swing upper body too fast. Breathe evenly. Keep weight in center.

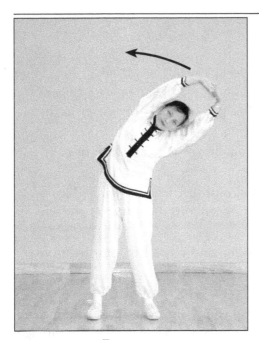

FIGURE 7-3

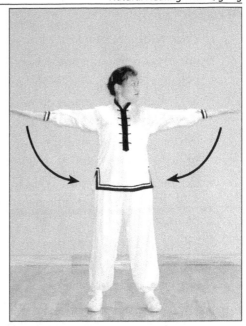

FIGURE 7-4

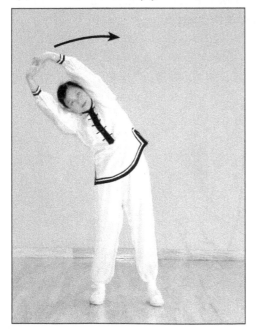

FIGURE 7-5

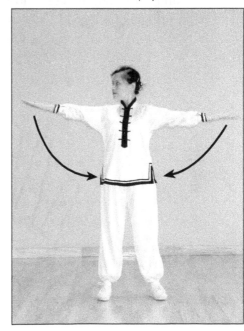

FIGURE 7-6

8 *"Tea pot" push*

1. Place your feet shoulder width apart.

2. Put fists on the side of the waist with palms up. Take deep breath.

3. Exhale and slowly turn body to the left pushing right hand forward (Figure 8-1). Left hand remains on waist like a "tea pot" shape. Focus energy in the center of the right hand.

4. Inhale and turn body back to front position, bring right hand back to waist, in fist position, palm up. (Figure 8-2)

5. Exhale and slowly turn body to right and push left hand forward. (Figure 8-3) Right hand remains on waist. Focus energy in the center of the left palm.

6. Inhale and turn body back to front position and move left hand back on waist.

7. Repeat above movements.

Important: Keep back straight when turning your waist, push hand with focused mind on palm energy, exhale as you push, all your negative energy is going out through the exhale and your Laogong point (in the center of the palm). Inhale when you bring hand back, bringing back good, smooth, and positive energy.

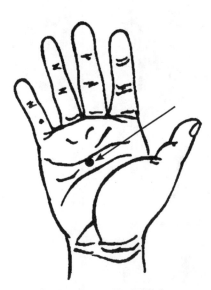

The Laogong (P-8) Cavity

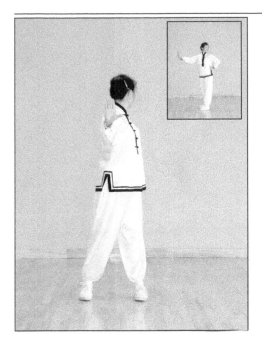

FIGURE 8-1

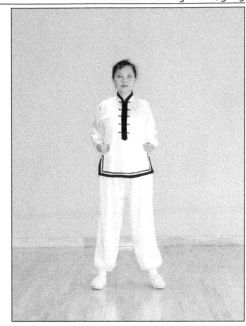

FIGURE 8-2

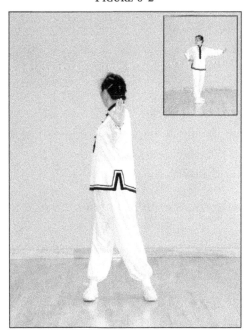

FIGURE 8-3

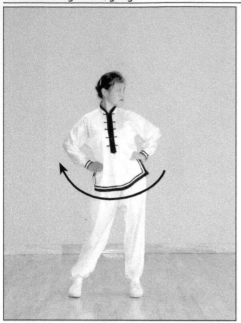

FIGURE 9-1   FIGURE 9-2

9 Hip rotation

1. Place your feet shoulder width apart.

2. Place hands on hips.

3. Slowly circle hip clockwise; left, forward, right, and back, 4 times. (Figure 9-1)

4. Slowly circle hip counter-clockwise; right, forward, left, and back, 4 times. (Figure 9-2)

Important: Legs and back are kept straight. Breathe evenly.

10 Arm raise and fly down

1. Step out to the left. Distance between feet is 1.5 of shoulder width.

2. Overlap hands (Figure 10-1), inhale slowly raising hands up above head with arms straight. (Figure 10-2)

3. Exhale and separate hands, until arms are straight on both sides at shoulder level, palms up, eyes follow left. (Figure 10-3)

4. Slowly bend upper body forward until body is at 90-degree angle to the legs, (arms are still outstretched to the sides). (Figure 10-4)

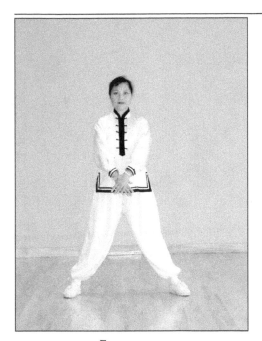

FIGURE 10-1

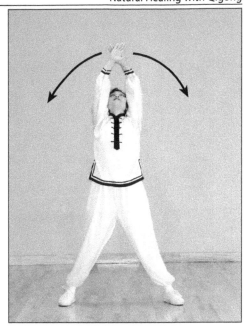

FIGURE 10-2

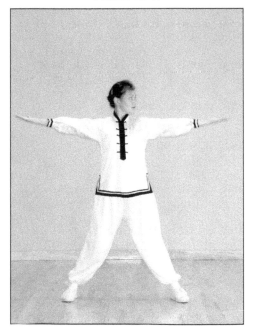

FIGURE 10-3

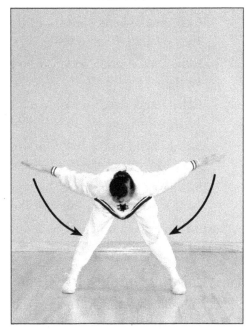

FIGURE 10-4

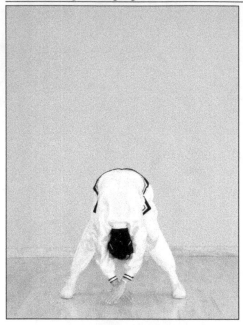

FIGURE 10-5

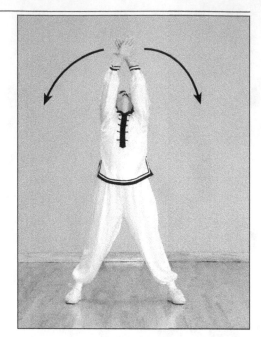

FIGURE 10-6

5. Continue to bend upper body down in the front and move hands down until they overlap. (Figure 10-5)

6. Inhale, raise arms and the body until your hands above the head, body straight. (Figure 10-6)

7. Exhale and separate hands to the side, with arms straight out at shoulder level, palms up, eyes follow right.

8. Slowly bend upper body forward until body is at a 90-degree angle to the legs. Move arms down and relax hands.

9. Slowly roll up the upper body one vertebrae at a time. Arms and hands are held loosely at your side and the knees are slightly bent.

Important: Keep arm and back straight at Step 6. Arms straight at steps 2, 3, 4, 6, and 7.

11 *Lunge position and stretch to side*

1. Stepping to the left, turn to the left and move straightened right hand forward to left, exhale. (Figure 11-1), Left fist is on the waist, bend left knee and keep right leg straight.

2. Turn your body back and shift your weight to center, legs straight, fists on waist, inhale. (Figure 11-2)

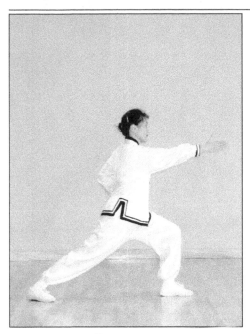

FIGURE 11-1

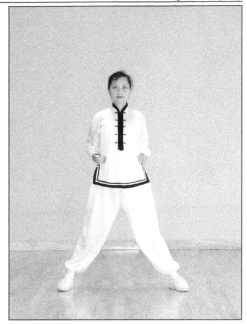

FIGURE 11-2

3. Turn body to right and move straightened left hand forward to right, exhale. Right fist on waist, bend right leg and keep left leg straight. (Figure 11-3

4. Turn your body back shifting weight to center with legs straight and fists on waist.

5. Repeat Steps 1 through 4.

6. Bring left foot back to center.

Important: When in the lunge position, remember to stretch hip to the maximum, keeping arms and back straight. Breathe evenly. Breathe out as you stretch out hand, breathe in as you move weight to center, hands on waist.

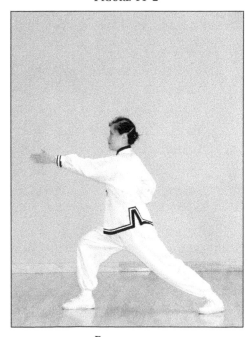

FIGURE 11-3

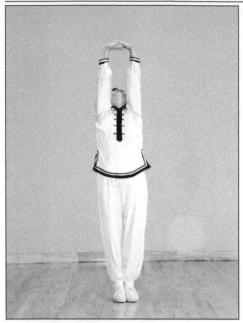

FIGURE 12-1   FIGURE 12-2

12 *Reach and touch feet*

1. Place your feet together.

2. Inhale, interlock fingers in front of the body and raise hands up above the head with palms upward, arms straight. (Figure 12-1)

3. Exhale, slowly bending forward, and then downward. Keep cervical and thoracic vertebrae straight along with your arm when you are bending down until reaching your feet, keep head relaxed, letting gravity gently stretch your head and head down. (Figure 12-2)

4. Release hands, and roll up gradually to starting position, keeping the body relaxed

Repeat Steps 2 through 4.

Important: Keep upper back straight when you are bending forward at Steps 2 and 3. Upper body and arms move together when bending forward and downward.

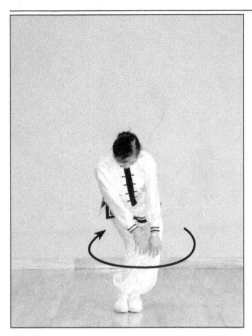

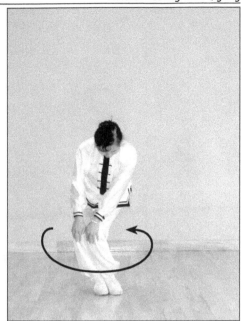

FIGURE 13-1

FIGURE 13-2

Group C.
Prevent and help to relieve hip, lower back and leg problems (disc problems, lower back muscle degeneration, hip joint and muscle degeneration or chronic injuries, arthritis).

13 *Knee rotation*

1. Place feet together.
2. Place both hands lightly on your knees.
3. Slowly circle knees clockwise 4 times. (Figure 13-1)
4. Then slowly circle knee opposite direction (counterclockwise) 4 times. (Figure 13-2)

Important: Circle knee as widely as you can. Breathe evenly.

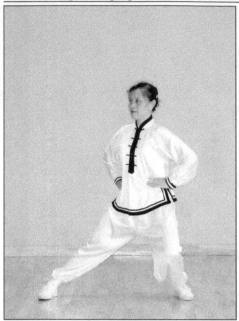

FIGURE 14-1   FIGURE 14-2

14 *Side lunge, turn body opposite 45 degrees*

1. Take a big step to the left and place both hands on waist

2. Slowly bend left leg and turn your body to the right side at a 45-degree angle, exhale. (Figure 14-1)

3. Slowly turn body back to center position, straightening both legs and putting weight in center, inhale.

4. Slowly bend right leg and turn body to the left side at a 45-degree angle, exhale. (Figure 14-2)

5. Slowly turn to center and straighten both legs, bring weight to center, inhale.

Repeat Steps 2 through 5.

Important: Bend legs as low as you can and keep back straight. As you are bending, turning, and raising the body, you may feel as if your Qi is sinking and rising.

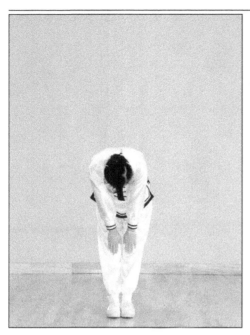

FIGURE 15-1

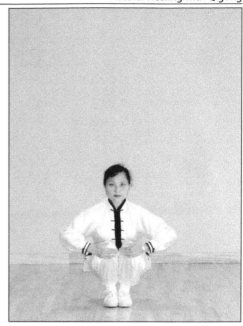

FIGURE 15-2

15 *Cover knee and stretch leg*

1. Place feet together.

2. Place both hands on knees. (Figure 15-1)

3. Slowly bend both knees while keeping good support from feet so you feel rooted. (Figure 15-2)

4. Place hands on the top of the feet, slowly raise hip as you straighten legs with hands on the top of feet. (Figure 15-3)

5. Slowly roll the upper body up and let hands relax at your side.

Repeat Steps 2 through 5.

Important: Normal breathing. Try to keep hands on feet as you raise hip and straighten legs.

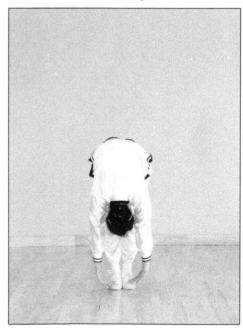

FIGURE 15-3

16 *Cover opposite knee and raise arm*

1. Step to the left, feet distance is 1.5 of shoulder width.

2. Bending forward and covering left knee with the right hand, while straightening the leg, inhale. (Figure 16-1)

3. Raise left arm forward and up over your head, keeping palm facing outward then upward, simultaneously bending both knees into horse riding position, exhale. (Figure 16-2)

4. Straighten legs and cover right knee with left hand, hands are on opposite knees, inhale. (Figure 16-3)

5. Raise right hand up, bending legs, and exhale.

6. Straighten legs and cover left knee with right hand (hands on opposite knees), inhale.

7. Raise left hand up, bending both knees into horse riding position, exhale. (Figure 16-4)

8. Straighten legs and cover right knee with left hand (hands on opposite knees), inhale.

9. Raise right hand up, bend legs and exhale.

Important: Breathe evenly. When in the horse riding position, keep your back straight and do not go beyond your comfort level.

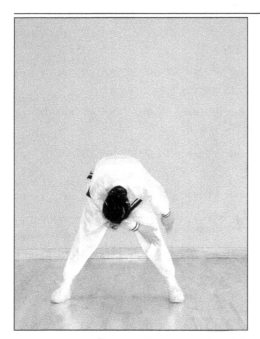

FIGURE 16-1

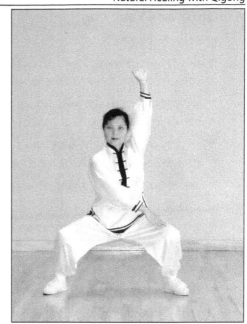

FIGURE 16-2

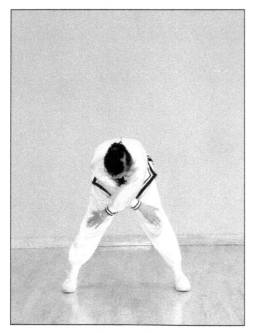

FIGURE 16-3

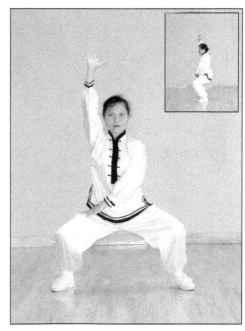

FIGURE 16-4

17 *Arm raise and knee hug*

1. Keep feet together.

2. Slowly step forward with left foot, putting weight on left foot, raise arms straight above head, palms inward, inhale. (Figure 17-1)

3. Separate arms to the side, lift up right knee (Figure 17-2) and hold with both hands as high as you can, exhale. (Figure 17-3)

4. Step back with right foot and raise arms up again with palm inward, arms straight, weight on left foot. (Figure 17-1)

5. Circle arms down to your side and step back with left foot.

6. Slowly step forward with right foot putting weight on right foot, raise arms straight above head, palm inward, inhale.

7. Separate arms to the side then lift left knee with hands as high as you can, exhale. (Figures 17-2 and 17-3)

8. Step back with left foot and raise arms above head again, palm inward, weight on right foot, inhale. (Figure 17-1)

9. Circle arms to side then down, step back right foot.

Important: Stretch arms as high as you can. Breathe deeply. Hold knee as close possible to your chest.

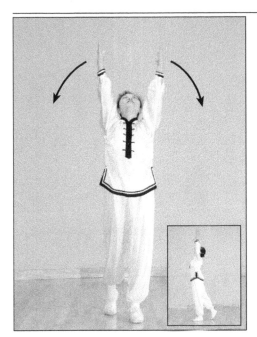

FIGURE 17-1

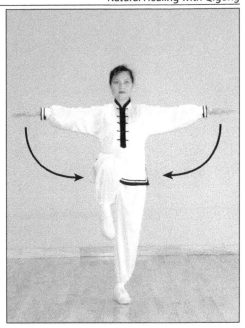

FIGURE 17-2

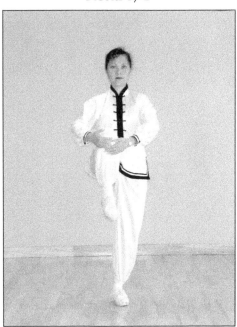

FIGURE 17-3

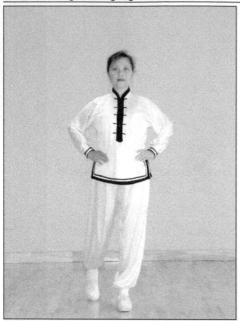

FIGURE 18-1   FIGURE 18-2

18 *Slow walking forward and backward*

1. Place feet together, place hands on waist, and relax shoulders.

2. Step forward with left foot (Figure 18-1), lift right heel, keeping weight on left foot.

3. Shift weight back to right foot (sit back, bend right knee), lift left toe up. (Figure 18-2)

4. Step forward with right foot and put weight on right, left heel up.

5. Shift weight to left leg (sit back, bending left knee), right toe up and heel down.

6. Shift weight to right foot with both legs straight, left heel up.

7. Again shift weight to left (sit back) and right toe up.

8. Step back with right foot.

9. Step back with left foot, bringing feet together.

10. Repeat above with opposite foot movement, step forward with right foot (Refer to Step 2).

Important: Walk slowly. When shifting weight, put full weight on one side then the other, keeping back straight. Breathe evenly. When stepping back, step with toe first, and the rest of the foot follows (toe, ball of the foot, heel). When steeping forward, heel down first then the ball of the foot, and finally the toe.

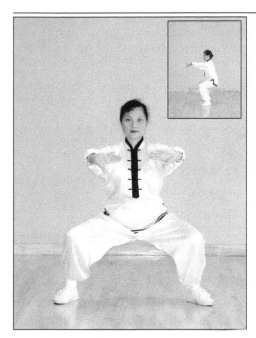

FIGURE 19-1

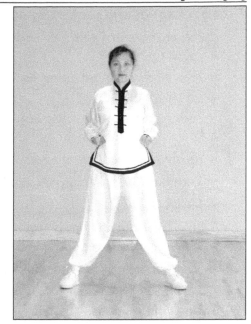

FIGURE 19-2

Section II

Group D
Help to relieve and prevent arms and leg ailments (arthritis, bursitis, tendonitis, muscle injury or degeneration).

19 Horse ride and push palm

1. Step to left, hands (fists) on waist, palms up, inhale.

2. Push both palms forward with fingers facing center, bending both legs, (horse riding position), exhale. (Figure 19-1)

3. Turn palms up and bring hands back onto waist, while straightening legs. (Figure 19-2)

4. Repeat above movements for a total of four times.

Important: Exhale as you push hands out. As you are exhaling, try to let everything uncomfortable or disturbing in your life go out through your arm and palm (Laogong point is in the center of the palm). When you bend leg in the horse riding position, keep your back straight.

20 *Turn back squat and push hand out*

1. Feet are separated with one fist distance between them, hands (fists) on waist, palms up.

2. Turn body left until facing back without moving the feet (but the feet do pivot around).

3. Push right hand and slowly bend both legs crossing your knees, turn head to left, left hand remains on waist. (Figure 20-1)

4. Slowly straighten legs and withdraw right hand back to waist.

5. Turn body back to center position hands (fists) on waist.

6. Turn body to the right until facing back without dislocation of feet.

7. Push left hand and slowly bend both legs crossing your knees, turn head to right, right hand remains on waist. (Figure 20-2)

8. Slowly straighten legs and withdraw left hand back on waist.

9. Turn body back to center position hands (fists) on waist.

Important: Keep back straight as you push hand and bend knees. Turn head (stretching neck) as far as you can. Exhale while pushing hand.

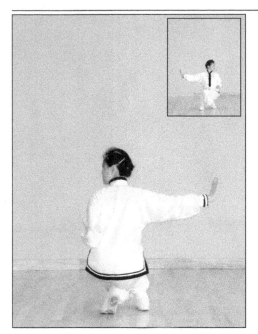

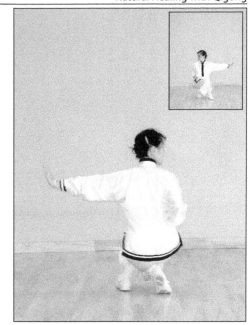

FIGURE 20-1

FIGURE 20-2

21 *Go through up and down*

1. Place feet together, hands (fists) on waist, palms up. (Figure 21-1)

2. Raise right hand up above head, arm straight and palm upward, inhale. (Figure 21-2)

3. Turn body to the left without moving feet. (Figure 21-3)

4. Exhale and slowly move right hand down along left side of the body (Figure 21-4) all the way to the feet then cross over feet. (Figure 21-5)

5. Inhale, continue moving right hand up along right side of your body then place right hand on waist, straighten body, and exhale. (You should feel that you are moving the energy through your body.)

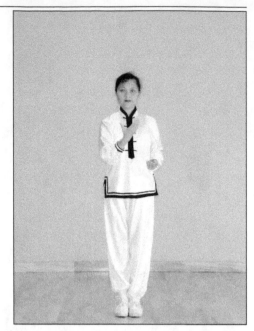

FIGURE 21-1

6. Raise left hand up above head, arm straight and palm up, inhale. (Opposite of Figure 21-2)

7. Turn body to right without moving feet. (Opposite of Figure 21-3)

8. Exhale and slowly move left hand down along right side of the body all the way to the feet. (Opposite of Figures 21-4 and 21-5)

9. Inhale, continue moving left hand up along left side of the body, place left hand back on waist, straighten body, and exhale.

Important: Feet together. Knees straight.

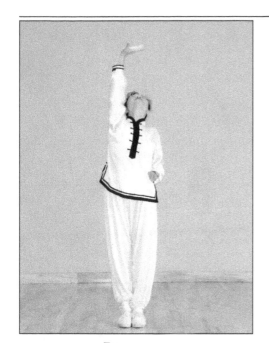

FIGURE 21-2

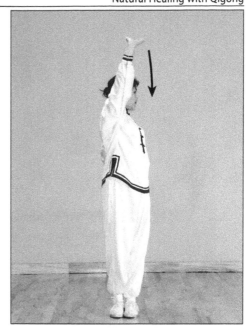

FIGURE 21-3

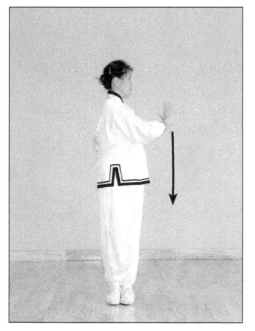

FIGURE 21-4

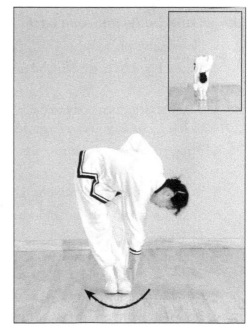

FIGURE 21-5

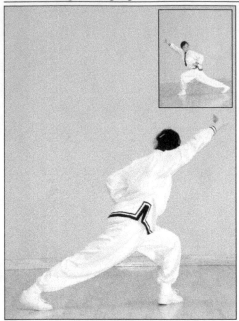

FIGURE 22-1

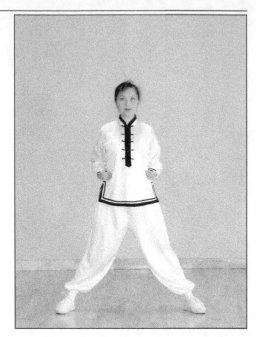

FIGURE 22-2

22 *Lunge, turn body, and look back*

1. Place hands on waist.

2. Take a big step to the left and turn the left foot to the left approximately 150 degrees.

3. Bend left leg, turn body to the left and push right hand to upper left and look to left as far as you can (right leg straight). (Figure 22-1)

4. Bring right hand back to waist, turn left toe to front, bring body to center position.(Figure 22-2)

5. Bring left foot together with right foot.

6. Take a big step to right and turn right foot to right 150 degrees. (Opposite of Figure 21-1)

7. Bend the right leg, turn body to right and push left hand to upper right and look to the right as far as you can (left leg straight). (Opposite of Figure 21-2)

8. Bring left hand back to waist and turn right toe to front, bring body to center position. (Opposite of Figures 21-3 and 21-4)

9. Bring right foot together with left foot.

Important: Turn body and lean forward as far as you can. In this movement, all parts of the body get a good stretching.

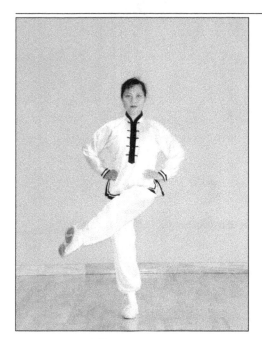

FIGURE 23-1   FIGURE 23-2

23 Alternate leg kick

1. Put both hands on waist.

2. Slowly raise left leg and kick to the right. (Figure 23-1)

3. Slowly raise right leg and kick to the left. (Figure 23-2)

4. Repeat Steps 2 and 3 for a total of four times.

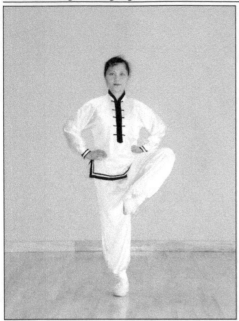

FIGURE 24-1 FIGURE 24-2

24 *Feet joggling*

1. Keep both hands on waist.

2. Kick up left foot with inner side of the foot. (Figure 24-1)

3. Kick up right foot with inner side of the foot. (Figure 24-2)

4. Kick up left foot with outer side of foot. (Figure 24-3)

5. Kick up right foot with outer side of foot. (Figure 24-4)

6. Kick forward with the left foot. (Figure 24-5)

7. Kick forward with the right foot.

8. Kick backward with the left foot, heel close to your gluteus region. (Figure 24-6)

9. Kick backward with the right foot, heel close to your gluteus region

Benefits: This is a good exercise for all joints on the lower part of the body. Doing it correctly can prevent arthritis, bursitis, and tendonitis.

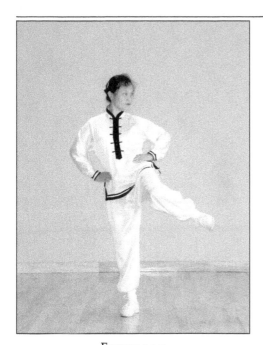

FIGURE 24-3

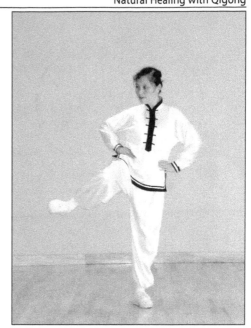

FIGURE 24-4

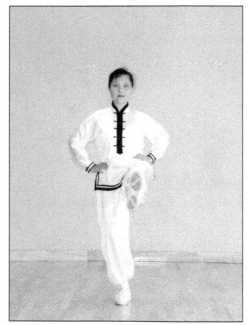

FIGURE 24-5

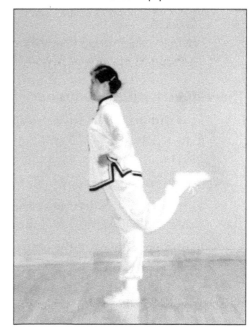

FIGURE 24-6

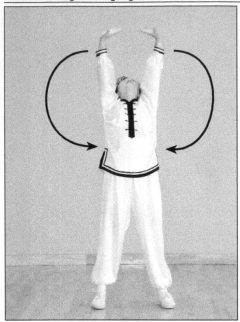

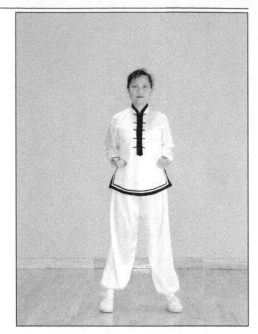

FIGURE 25-1   FIGURE 25-2

Group E.
Help to relieve and prevent illness in area of hands, wrist, elbow
(tendonitis in wrist, elbow and hands).

25 *Three-direction push hands out*

1. Start with feet shoulder width apart.

2. Raise hands up above your head, arms straight and palms up, inhale. (Figure 25-1)

3. Bring arms sideways down, fists to waist and exhale. (Figure 25-2)

4. Turn body to the left, raise hands up to chest level, then push hands out (front and backward), and inhale. (Figures 25-3 and 25-4)

5. Return upper body to the center and bring hands (fists) back onto waist and exhale. (Figure 25-2)

6. Turn body to the right, push hands out (front and backward), and inhale. (Figure 25-5)

7. Bring hands (fists) back onto waist and exhale. (Figure 25-2)

8. Stay in center position and push hands to side, inhale (Figure 25-6).

9. Bring hands back onto waist and exhale. (Figure 25-2)

Important: Do not move feet when turning waist. Keep back straight.

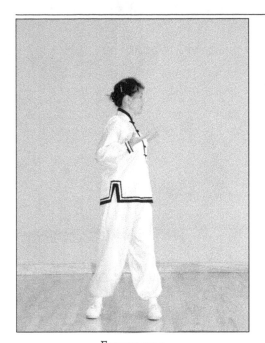

FIGURE 25-3

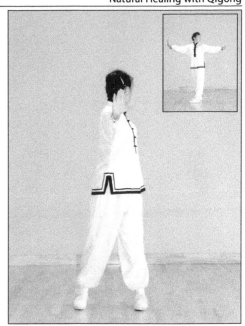

FIGURE 25-4

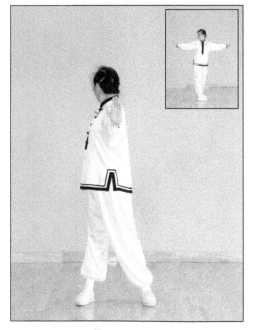

FIGURE 25-5

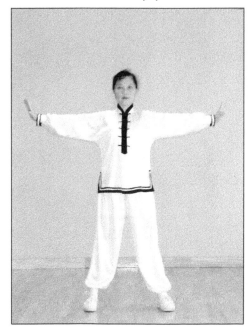

FIGURE 25-6

26 *Shooting Arrow*

1. Take a big step to the left. Cross wrists in the front, inhale. (Figure 26-1)

2. Bending both knees, push left hand to the left, change right hand to a fist and pull to the right as if you were pulling back an arrow but with palm (fist) down, exhale. (Figure 26-2)

3. Bring hands to front at chest level and press down with palm, straightening both legs and inhale. (Figure 26-3)

4. Bring left foot back to the center and exhale.

5. Step to the right, crossing hands in front and inhale. (Figure 26-1)

6. Bending knees, push right hand to the right, left hand makes a fist and pulls back as if you are pulling back an arrow but palm down, exhale. (Opposite of Figure 26-2)

7. Bring hands to the front and press down while straightening legs and inhale.

8. Bring right foot back and exhale. (Figure 26-3)

Important: Keep back straight when bending both legs. Keep arm straight when pushing hand, eyes follow the hand that is pushing.

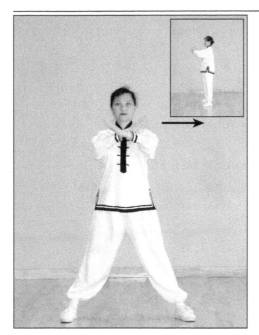

FIGURE 26-1

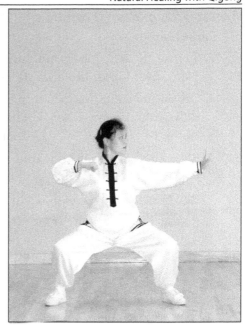

FIGURE 26-2

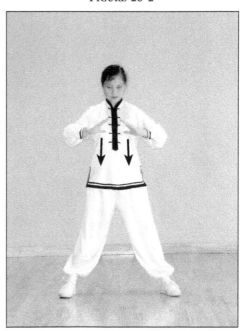

FIGURE 26-3

27 Arm stretch and wrist rotation

Part One:

1. Step to the left, inhale and raise hands up with arms straight, palm facing palm. Eyes follow hands up. (Figure 27-1)

2. Exhale and make fists then turn fists outward, rotate arms and wrists sideways down to waist, eyes follow left hand then return to the center. The body does not move. (Figures 27-2, 27-3, and 27-4)

3. Raise hands up again with arms straight, same as Step 1.

4. Exhale and make fists then turn fists outward, rotate arms and wrists sideways down to waist, eyes follow right hand then return to the center.

5. Repeat all of the above steps.

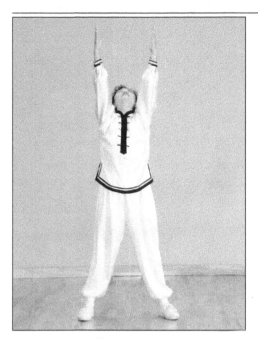

FIGURE 27-1

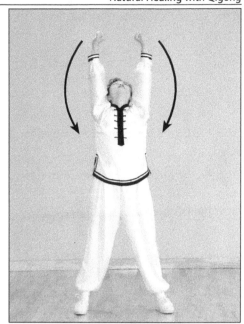

FIGURE 27-2

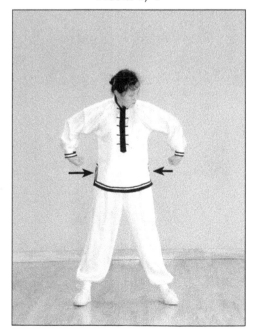

FIGURE 27-3

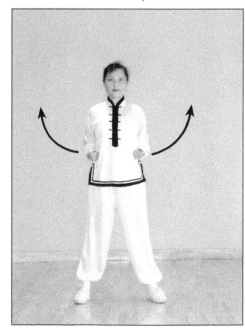

FIGURE 27-4

Arm stretch and wrist rotation

Part Two:

1. Feet stay same as above. Inhale, extend arms downward, and back to the sides of your body, raise arms until they are over your head, palms inward. Eyes follow right side up.

2. Exhale, make fists and move fists down in front of your body to the lower torso. Eyes follow hands down. (Figures 27-5, 27-6, and 27-7)

3. Inhale, extend arms downward and backward, raise arms back and up until overhead, palms inward. Eyes follow left side up (refer to Step 1 in Part Two).

4. Exhale, repeat Step 2 in Part Two

5. Repeat above.

Important: Extend arms as wide as you can. Rotate all of the joints in the arms. Breathe deeply and slowly follow the movements.

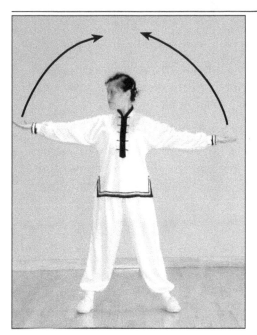

FIGURE 27-5

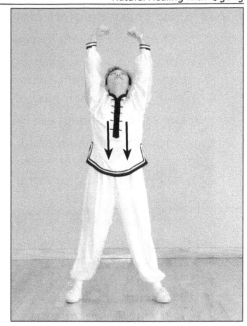

FIGURE 27-6

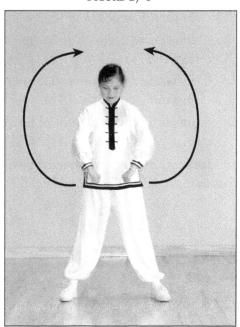

FIGURE 27-7

28 *Forward and backward stretching*

1. Place feet together, both fists on waist.

2. Push right hand up and forward, rotate left fist inward and backward, arms straight, keep waist still, rotate only the joints of the shoulder, elbow, and wrist. Eyes look back towards the left hand. (Figure 28-1)

3. Rotate wrists and bring both hands back to waist, in fist position.

4. Push left hand up and forward, rotate right fist inward and backward, arms straight, keep waist still, rotate only the joints of the shoulder, elbow, and wrist. Eyes look back towards the right hand and bring hands back on waist. (Opposite of Figure 28-1)

5. Repeat above steps for a total of 4 times.

Important: Keep body straight up, do not turn waist, keep shoulders still, only work on joints in neck, shoulder, elbow, and wrists.

29 *Horse ride boxing*

1. Take a wide step to the left. Place both fists on waist and take a deep breath

2. Exhale and slowly punch forward with left fist while bending both legs in horse riding position. (Figure 29-1)

3. Inhale and turn left palm up withdraw left hand back to waist, straighten legs.

4. Exhale and slowly punch forward with right fist and bend legs in horse riding position.

5. Inhale and turn right palm up and bring hand back to waist (fist).

6. Repeat all the steps 4 times.

Important: Keep back straight when punching forward with fists. When punching forward, extend until arm is straight.

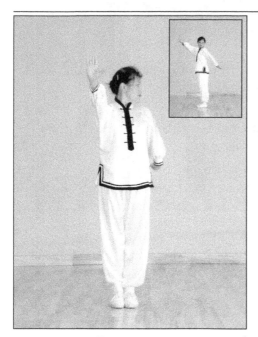

FIGURE 28-1

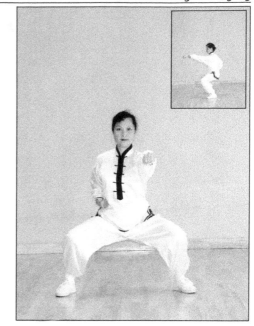

FIGURE 29-1

30 *Swing arm and upper body*

1. Place feet shoulder width apart.

2. Turn upper body and swing arms to the left, placing right hand on the left shoulder, left hand goes to the right waist, palm facing out. (Figure 30-1 and 30-2)

3. Turn upper body and swing arms to the right, left hand goes to the right shoulder, right hand on left waist, palm facing out. (Figure 30-3 and 30-4)

4. Repeat 2 and 3 for total of 4 times. Relax whole body.

Important: Do not move your feet when you turn your body and swing your arms. Turn body and head in the same direction, as far as you can. Eyes follow in the same direction you turn your body.

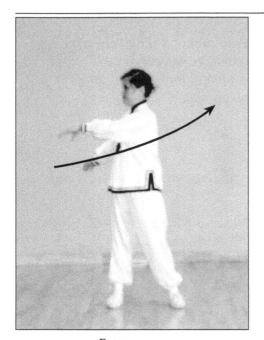

FIGURE 30-1

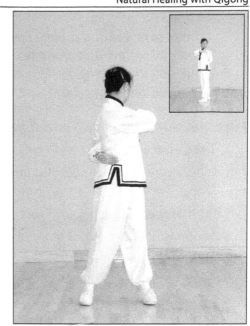

FIGURE 30-2

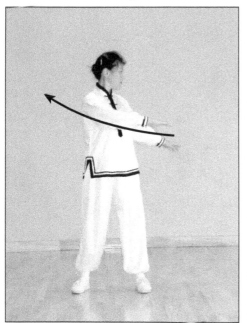

FIGURE 30-3

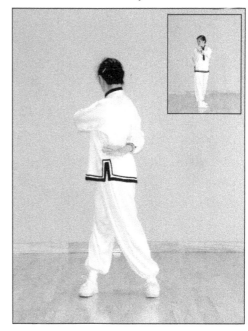

FIGURE 30-4

Group F.
Helps to relieve and prevent illness in internal organs, strengthens internal organs, and promotes energy circulation. Prevents aging. Alleviates hypertension, heart disease, gastrointestinal diseases, stress, anxiety, low energy, headache, and nasal congestion.

31 Face, massage, and hand massage

1. Face massage

Use index or middle finger to massage on the acupressure points. Follow the points:

Corner of mouth. Dichang. (Figure 31-1)

Side of nostril. Yanxiang. (Figure 31-2)

Middle of the nose at indent point. Bitong (Figure 31-3)

At beginning of the eyebrow, close to center of nose. Zanzhu (Figure 31-4)

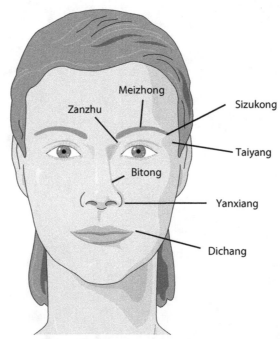

THESE SEVEN POINTS ON THE FACE HELP TO RELIEVE COMMON COLDS, HEADACHE, SINUS PROBLEMS, RELAX FACIAL MUSCLES, AND RELIEVE STRESS

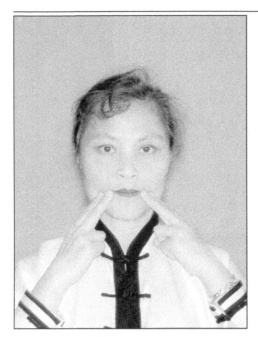

FIGURE 31-1

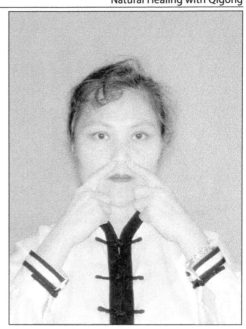

FIGURE 31-2

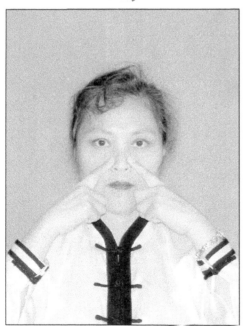

FIGURE 31-3

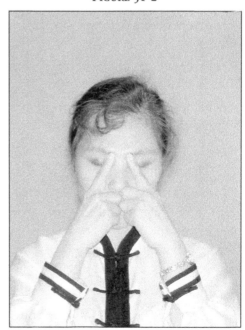

FIGURE 31-4

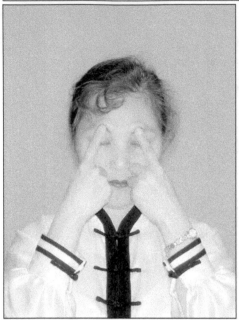

FIGURE 31-5

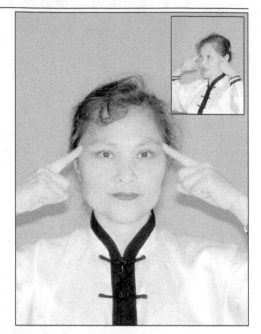

FIGURE 31-6

In the middle of the eyebrow. Meizhong (Figure 31-5)

At the end of the eyebrow. Sizukong (Figure 31-6)

Temple point in the depression area. Taiyang (Figure 31-7)

2. Head Massage

Use thumb, starting at the front ear lobe (Figure 31-8), to gradually push up while the rest of the fingers press on the head (Figure 31-9); slowly massage downward while the thumb behind the ear massages downward (Figures 31-10 and 31-11).

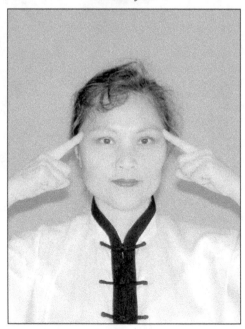

FIGURE 31-7

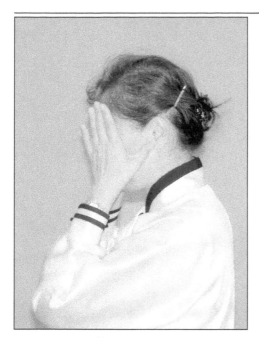

FIGURE 31-8

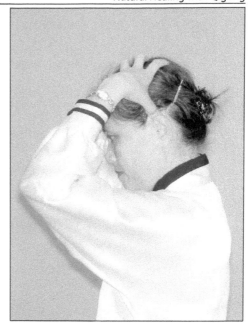

FIGURE 31-9

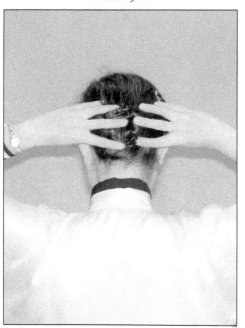

FIGURE 31-10

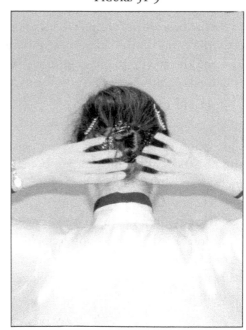

FIGURE 31-11

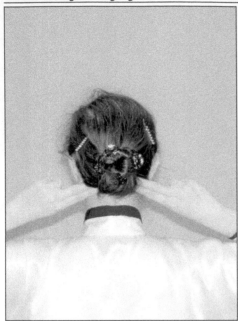

FIGURE 31-12

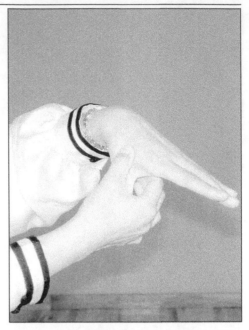

FIGURE 31-13

At the base of the scalp, 1.5 inches from centerline on both sides, use forefinger and middle finger to massage these areas. (Figure 31-12)

3. Hand massage

Use thumb and index finger to massage the opposite hand at the corner between thumb and index metacarpal bone, one inch away from the wedge. (Figures 31-13 and 31-14)

Benefits: Relieves headaches, migraines, common colds, nasal congestion, high stress, anxiety, eye discomfort, poor vision, stiff neck, poor memory, drooling, and insomnia.

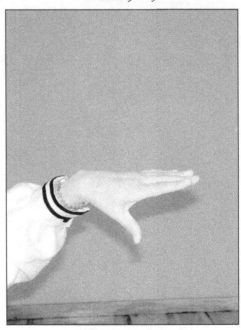

FIGURE 31-14

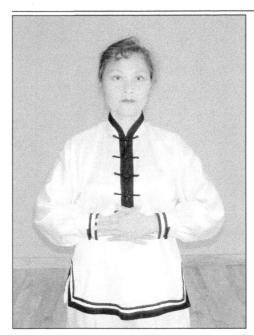

FIGURE 32-1   FIGURE 32-2

32 *Abdominal massage*

1. Overlap the palms (male left hand under right hand, female right hand under left hand).

2. Massage upper abdomen clockwise 4 times. (Figure 32-1)

3. Massage whole abdomen clockwise 4 times. (Figure 32-2)

4. Massage whole abdomen 4 times counterclockwise.

5. Massage upper abdomen 4 times counterclockwise.

Benefits: Relieves stomach pain, nausea, bloated stomach, poor digestion, lower abdominal pain, cramps and discomfort, constipation, and diarrhea. Useful for soothing a baby who cries at night.

33 *Hair combing and scalp massage*

1. Place feet shoulder width apart.

2. Inhale, put left hand behind your back, using your right hand (fingers) massage scalp, start at top center, comb back along the middle line of your head. (Figure 33-1)

3. Exhale, turn upper body to the left as you continue to comb down. (Figure 33-2)

4. Use right hand to massage left side of neck. (Figure 33-3)

5. Turn body back to center and massage right temple point (Taiyang point). (Figure 33-4)

6. Inhale, put right hand behind your back. Using left hand (fingers), massage scalp. (Similar to Step 2).

7. Turn body to the right as you continue to massage downward.

8. Massage right side of neck (with left hand).

9. Turn body back to center and massage left temple point.

Important: Should be done on a regular basis.

Benefits: Relieves headaches, backaches, migraines, dizziness, insomnia, stiff neck and other neck and shoulder problems, improves memory and relieves stress.

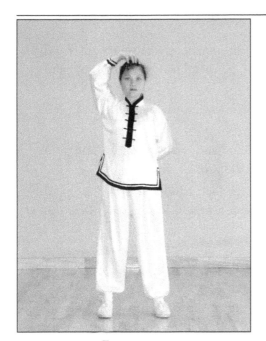

FIGURE 33-1

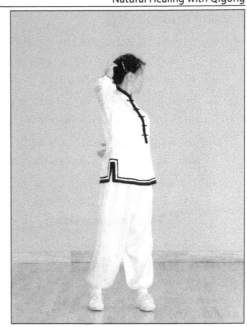

FIGURE 33-2

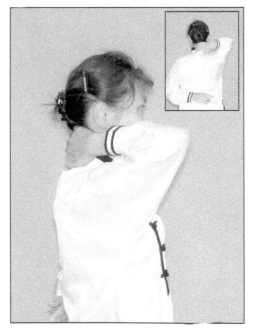

FIGURE 33-3

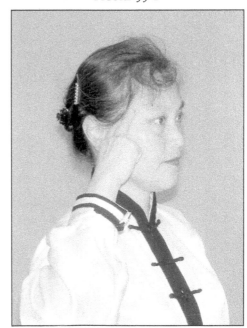

FIGURE 33-4

34 *Raising arm and leg*

1. Put weight on right leg, raise left knee, simultaneously raising right hand above head with palm up and arm straight, left hand is next to the hip, palm facing down. (Figure 34-1)

2. Slowly step down with your left foot, press down with the right hand, left hand turn palm up. (Figure 34-2)

3. Raise right leg, simultaneously raising left hand with palm up and arm straight, let right hand gentle press down. (Figure 34-3)

4. Step down with right foot, pressing down with left hand and turn right hand palm up. (Figure 34-4) Inhale when raising arm and leg, exhale when you press down and step down.

5. Repeat above.

Important: Breathing deeply and slowly, raise arm as high as you can, and press opposite hand as low as you can.

Benefits: Relieves dizziness, poor balance, fatigue, shortness of breath, poor digestion, stomach ache, diarrhea, body ache, etc.

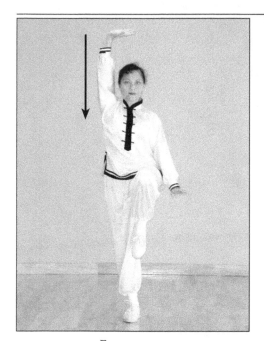

FIGURE 34-1

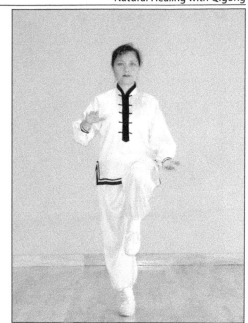

FIGURE 34-2

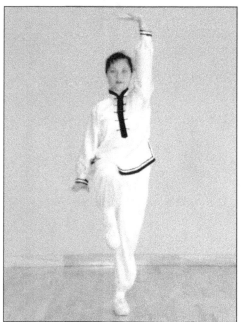

FIGURE 34-3

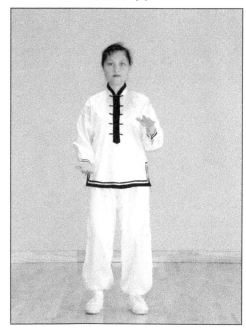

FIGURE 34-4

35 *Four-direction movements*

1. Take a big step to the left.

2. Raise both hands up above your head and turn palms up. (Figure 35-1)

3. Bring hands down over lower back to support the back. (Figure 35-2, 35-3)

4. Turn waist left, 90 degrees. (Figure 35-4)

5. Turn waist right, 90 degrees. (Figure 35-5)

6. Return to center.

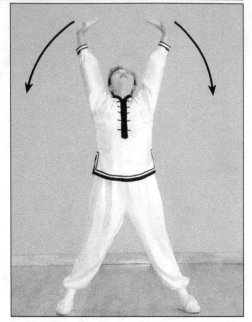

FIGURE 35-1

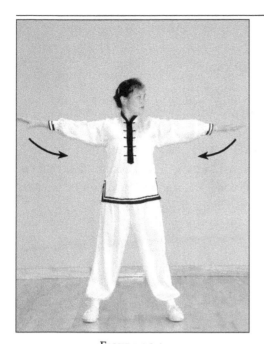

FIGURE 35-2

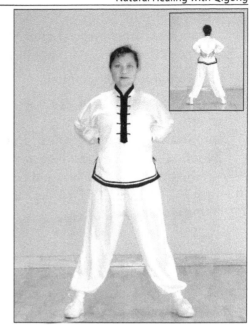

FIGURE 35-3

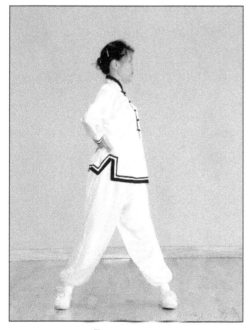

FIGURE 35-4

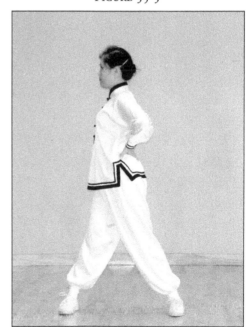

FIGURE 35-5

7. Slowly bend forward as low as you can, keeping your back straight and let your head drop down. (Figure 35-6)

8. Raise body and head up, and then bend backwards. (Figure 35-7)

9. Return to a center position.

10. Repeat above movements, however, at Step 4 turn to the right and Step 5 turn to the left.

Important: Breathing deeply and slowly, stretch and bend body as far as you can.

Benefits: Improves digestive system, strengthens kidney and back muscles, relieves degeneration of spinal vertebra, and backache. Good for fatigue, weak kidney energy, dizziness, eye problems, and ringing ear. Improves energy level.

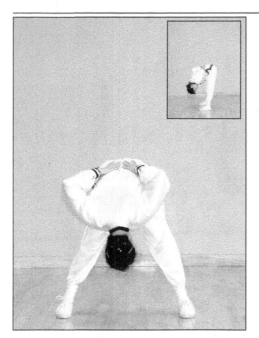

FIGURE 35-6

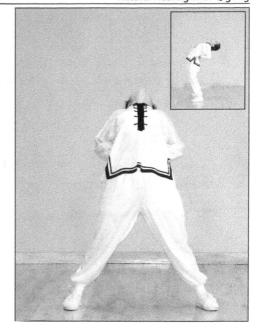

FIGURE 35-7

36 Arm raise and deep breathing

1. Place feet shoulder width apart.

2. Slowly raise hands in front going up as high as you can (slightly lifting your heels if you choose), inhale. (Figure 36-1)

3. Slowly lower both hands, and exhale. (Figure 36-2, 36-3)

4. Repeat Steps 2 and 3 for a total of four times. Breathe deeply at each movement.

5. Take deep breath and relax whole body. (Figure 36-4)

Benefits: Improves cardiovascular and respiratory functions. Increases energy level. Relieves stress.

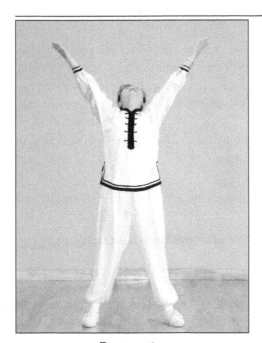

FIGURE 36-1

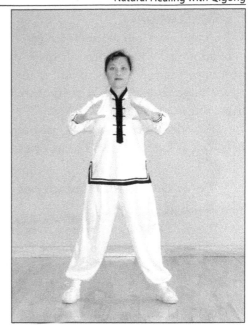

FIGURE 36-2

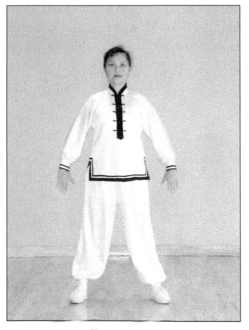

FIGURE 36-3

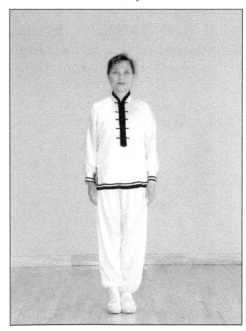

FIGURE 36-4

CONCLUSION

Qigong is a gift from 4000 years of Chinese culture that gives us many health benefits we take for granted. It helps us to not only prevent illness and strengthen the immune system, but also to heal many chronic illnesses. We can prevent many unnecessary surgeries and drug toxicity if we focus on Qigong practice at earlier stages of our lives. But it is never too late.

In modern society with its fast-paced life style, we need Qigong to slow us down to balance our lives and avoid heart disease in the future.

- We need Qigong to reduce our stress and lead us to more enjoyment in our lives.
- We need Qigong to help us to be more focused and avoid mistakes in our lives and at work.
- We need Qigong to help us grow our mind and wisdom.
- We need Qigong to help us to avoid mental disturbance and physical problems.
- We need Qigong to help us build a better life.

It is not too late to study at any age. Start today; start your healing and journey to health. Start to build a powerful mind, body, and life. Start to work on yourself and chose this path for your future to see what will happen in your life. Your diligent study of Qigong will be rewarding

Have a wonderful practice!

Students and Patients Speak

Several of my students and patients have written about their experiences with Qigong practice and with Chinese Medicine in my clinic. In this section, I have included excerpts from their letters. The students and patients are all Westerners who have chosen to explore the 4000-year-old Chinese way to health.

Qigong practice has helped to make me a more relaxed, healthy, and patient person. I find it essential in maintaining a healthy stress level in our hectic society. At this time, I am also fortunate to be teaching this exercise to others and witnessing the state of relaxation others achieve through practice.

— Jeanne M. (Cohasset)

When I first came to see Dr. Aihan Kuhn, I had been sick for two years. Recovering from a hysterectomy, I had many complications, anxiety, depression, urinary tract infections, yeast, and bacterial infections. Eight months before that, I had a breast biopsy. My headaches and fatigue were terrible and I had constant panic attacks. I did not know what else to do and my doctors were going no where with me, but giving me more antibiotics, which made me worse.

Dr. Aihan Kuhn…did acupressure on my ear immediately I felt better. She sent me home with tea to make and drink for a week. After that week, I felt better. Weeks later, she did acupuncture on my bladder and I am doing quite well. I have also had acupuncture on my back for arthritis and the pain and swelling are almost gone. …I have also learned Taiji and Qigong. These classes require much hard work because you must practice a lot. Nevertheless, it is a lot of fun and very rewarding.

I never dreamed I could learn Taiji, but everyone in the classes I took were so helpful and gave me so much encouragement. My first class was stressful because I was so scared. My hands and knees were shaking so hard I remember saying to myself "I am so nervous, how can I even learn this, this is impossible?" But everyone in the class said to me "do not stop trying, you'll get it, it takes time and practice." Okay I said and I practiced every day, every week for weeks and finally one week I got it. It just clicked in and I did it. I did Taiji! I was so proud of myself and so thankful for meeting such wonderful people who helped me and gave me all this encouragement.

Now I do Taiji and Qigong morning and night. It keeps me in balance and very healthy. I have more energy and less pain and disease….Alternative medicine, Dr. Aihan Kuhn and many people in her classes have helped me tremendously in my healing…

—Mary J.

I arrived on your doorstep in agony the day after I was told by a neurosurgeon that I'd have to have brain surgery ("a decompression") to alleviate the pressure of the fluid in my skull. I'd had brain surgery (shunt) twice before, and was not convinced this would solve my problem. I was in a lot of pain; could not walk, or even sit for any length of time…

Your "intensive care" program included herbal pills, Qigong, and healing massage… After 9 months, the head pain is no longer an issue. I have more energy, less depression, and feel kind of "normal" (I just get ordinary aches and pains)—it's so cool.

—Amy M.

I am a seventy-two year old woman who has been a participant in Oriental exercise classes taught by Aihan Kuhn once weekly for approximately a year and have found them to be good for my physical and mental well-being.

Since the exercises are enjoyable as well as beneficial, I do them on my own a t home between classes. I consider the time to be very well spent. The benefits are achieved without the necessity of quick, jerky movements and over-strenuous activity. There is no possibility for injury because of the teacher's caring and attention to each student's needs.

Specific benefits that I've experienced are increased vitality and flexibility resulting in fewer aches and pains that are a part of the aging process. It is wonderful to seldom have a back or headache. Very importantly stress-reduction for me has occurred naturally, creating physical and mental harmony…

—Marilyn B.

At the end of the exercise class, my mind and body feel so relaxed. I concentrate solely on what I am doing.

The exercises help all parts of my body from top of my head to my feet. And I must tell you it also helps to keep my blood pressure down.

Your classes…keep our bodies in shape and alleviate some of our bodily pains.

—Wanda M.

…I've always tried to be positive, because the way I see it, things go better from you when your positive, your body feels lighter. When your negative things do not go as well and your body feels much heavier. It takes fewer muscles to smile than to frown. When you feel good about yourself, you can make the people around you feel good too. A little smile goes a long way. I know the Qigong exercises have made me so far a calmer person not so nervous…. I enjoy the Qigong classes and plan on taking more. I enjoy the meetings I think I can learn a lot from them and it's nice just to be around such nice people. I know if I keep doing the Qigong exercises I can stay healthy, grow old gracefully, and be happy.

—Charlene B.

I will like to start this letter by saying how much I enjoyed Dr. Kuhn's **Therapeutic Qigong** seminar. Her enthusiasm for the practice of Qigong and her ability to project that enthusiasm was inspirational in and of itself. I hope that the seminar was the beginning of a long personal relationship with Chinese medicine.

—Nancy D.

I am 84 years old and Qigong is part of my life. I tell everyone about it and most people do not know what it is. For many years, I have watched the people of China do their exercises out in the parks and many of them are old people. I think of myself, and how good I feel. Some mornings I do not feel too well and I feel like skipping them, but I talk myself out of feeling sorry for myself and I put on the music tape. The music calms me and I get to work. I have not mastered the deep breathing yet. I know that when you breathe deeply your brain gets more oxygen and that helps you think more clearly.

I think that if you do your exercises in the open air like on the town common, people will take notice and become interested. People are curious and when they hear the music, they will stop and see what is going on.

We in America are all out of shape. Most workers just sit at a desk all day. I myself, when I worked as a welder, just sat at my machine all day. The only exercise I got was working my hands.

I think industry should lay aside some time for a little workout to change the positions and breathe new life into our robotic souls.

Qigong could be taught in schools in the gym class…

Now I am busy nearly every day and I tell my friends that I keep moving so the Grim Reaper will not know where I am.

—Jessica H.

I am 42 years old and had suffered from fibromyalgia for 5 years. I was in a lot of pain every day. I'm now feeling much better. I have much less pain and much more energy as the result of practicing **Therapeutic Qigong**.

—Donna W.

Since my introduction to **Therapeutic Qigong**, I have become convinced that it is an outstanding form of exercise for improving and maintaining general health and well-being. The benefits of its practice experienced personally included immune system function, greater flexibility, and range of motion, breathing capacity, and balance. With regular and diligent practice, I have found this form can help to increase the quality of sleep and elevate the spirit. I have also used it both before and after hard physical exertion to help prevent damage to muscle and joints.

—Steve L.

Final Words

Self-care or self-healing practice can make a big difference in the quality of your life. Self-healing therapies are not secondary. They are the most important part of any journey toward wholeness. You cannot arrive there unless you bring yourself along. Let your spirit guide you as you search for your path. Healing will follow.

I believe if you put enough effort on what you want to achieve, you should have no problem to get what you want. From my own experience, I got what I need and what I want through my hard work on Qigong practice.

I hope that Therapeutic Qigong will help you along your way.

Dr. Aihan Kuhn
C.M.D, DIPL. OBT,
Master of Tai Chi, Qigong
Director of Chinese Medicine
    for Health
President, Tai Chi & Qi Gong
    Healing Institute
Chinese Medicine for Health, Inc.
1564A Washington St.
Holliston, MA 01746
508-429-3895
www.taichihealing.com

Recommended Reading

BOOKS

Beinfield, Harriet and Korngold, Efrem. 1992. *Between Heaven and Earth. A Guide to Chinese Medicine*. New York: Ballantine Wellspring (Random House, Inc.). Clear explanations to help the beginner understand Chinese medicine.

Douglas, Bill. 1998. *The Complete Idiot's Guide to T'ai Chi and Qigong*. New York, NY: Alpha Books. An excellent book for beginners who have never been exposed to Taiji and Qigong.

Kuhn, Aihan. 2003. *Tai Chi Student Handbook. Chinese Medicine for Health*. Holliston, MA: New England School of Tai Chi.

Reid, Daniel. 1994. *The Complete Book of Chinese Health and Healing. Guarding the Three Treasures*. Boston, MA: Shambhala. Helpful for Westerners trying to understand the Chinese style of healing.

Yang, Jwing-Ming. 1997. *The Root of Chinese Qigong*. Boston, MA: YMAA Publication Center. For people who really want to explore the true nature of Qigong.

PERIODICALS

Qi Journal

Empty Vessel

Index

About the Author

Dr. Aihan Kuhn graduated in 1982 from the Hunan Medical University in Changsha, China. She trained in both conventional Western and Traditional Chinese Medicine (TCM). TCM is a natural healing medicine involving many different natural methods to treat various diseases. TCM can correct and balance the body's energy systems. For six years prior to coming to the United States in 1989, Dr Kuhn practiced medicine in a hospital in China as an obstetrician and gynecologist. In her practice, she was able to use both Western and Chinese Medicine. Since she was ten years old, she has been interested in Chinese Martial Arts and has studied sword 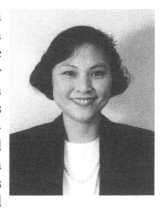 exercise. She has always been interested in nature and natural cures for illnesses. In 1978, she started to study Qigong, Taiji, and other oriental exercises. She began teaching these arts in China in 1984 and in the United States since 1992.

Dr Kuhn, who continues her study of Taiji and Qigong in China every year, has been mentored by well known Taiji and Qigong grand masters, such as Master Feng Zhi Qiang, a famous grand master of Chen style Taijiquan, and Duan Zhi Liang, a famous Qigong grand master and doctor. Her studies and explorations has sustained her high quality of teaching and helped her become more effective in her patient care and Chinese healing.

Dr. Kuhn believes that maintaining good health and preventing illness is more important than treating disease. To achieve a healthy lifestyle, Dr. Kuhn believes that one should work hard on improving Qi, the life force that is within us. She focuses on healthy ways of thinking and eating, routine Chinese exercise to enhance energy flow, and the practice of TCM to help others become well. To share her knowledge and experience in ancient Chinese healing, Dr. Kuhn has provided many on-site workshops and seminars to hospital professionals, wellness centers, senior centers, schools and colleges, nursing homes, and companies. Periodic lectures, as well as CEU programs for nurses and physical therapists, are held in her clinic. Dr. Kuhn has been teaching Taiji, Qigong, and other healing exercises in the United States since 1992. She is a Natural Psychologist who searches for wisdom from nature and applies it to daily life.

Dr. Kuhn is a Massachusetts state sponsor for the World Tai Chi and Qigong Day, an international event created to promote and foster awareness of the health benefits of practicing Taiji and Qigong. Taiji and Qigong groups all over the world go out and practice in public parks on the same day at same hour, to spread the healing spirit.

Dr. Kuhn is the director and owner of Chinese Medicine for Health, and President and founder of the Tai Chi & Qi Gong Healing Institute (TQHI). The latter is a non-profit organization that promotes natural energy healing and performs research with Qigong on diseases for which Western medicine has no cure. The main goal is to provide access to an improved quality of life. TQHI is committed to improving health care using traditional Chinese healing arts such as Qigong, Taiji, and other TCM methods to improve body energy circulation in order to heal many ailments, prevent illness, bring harmony to our society, and delay the aging process.

BOOKS FROM YMAA

more products available from . . .

YMAA Publication Center, Inc. 楊氏東方文化出版中心

1-800-669-8892 • info@ymaa.com • www.ymaa.com

BOOKS FROM YMAA (continued)

TAI CHI WALKING	B23X
TAIJI CHIN NA	B378
TAIJI SWORD—CLASSICAL YANG STYLE	B744
TAIJIQUAN THEORY OF DR. YANG, JWING-MING	B432
TENGU—THE MOUNTAIN GOBLIN	B1231
THE WAY OF KATA	B0584
THE WAY OF KENDO AND KENJITSU	B0029
THE WAY OF SANCHIN KATA	B0845
THE WAY TO BLACK BELT	B0852
TRADITIONAL CHINESE HEALTH SECRETS	B892
TRADITIONAL TAEKWONDO	B0665
WESTERN HERBS FOR MARTIAL ARTISTS	B1972
WILD GOOSE QIGONG	B787
WISDOM'S WAY	B361
XINGYIQUAN, 2ND ED.	B416

DVDS FROM YMAA

ADVANCED PRACTICAL CHIN NA IN-DEPTH	D1224
ANALYSIS OF SHAOLIN CHIN NA	D0231
BAGUAZHANG 1, 2, & 3—EMEI BAGUAZHANG	D0649
CHEN STYLE TAIJIQUAN	D0819
CHIN NA IN-DEPTH COURSES 1—4	D602
CHIN NA IN-DEPTH COURSES 5—8	D610
CHIN NA IN-DEPTH COURSES 9—12	D629
EIGHT SIMPLE QIGONG EXERCISES FOR HEALTH	D0037
ESSENCE OF TAIJI QIGONG	D0215
FIVE ANIMAL SPORTS	D1106
KUNG FU BODY CONDITIONING	D2085
KUNG FU FOR KIDS	D1880
NORTHERN SHAOLIN SWORD —SAN CAI JIAN, KUN WU JIAN, QI MEN JIAN	D1194
QIGONG MASSAGE	D0592
QIGONG FOR LONGEVITY	D2092
SABER FUNDAMENTAL TRAINING	D1088
SANCHIN KATA—TRADITIONAL TRAINING FOR KARATE POWER	D1897
SHAOLIN KUNG FU FUNDAMENTAL TRAINING—COURSES 1 & 2	D0436
SHAOLIN LONG FIST KUNG FU—BASIC SEQUENCES	D661
SHAOLIN LONG FIST KUNG FU—INTERMEDIATE SEQUENCES	D1071
SHAOLIN LONG FIST KUNG FU—ADVANCED SEQUENCES	D2061
SHAOLIN SABER—BASIC SEQUENCES	D0616
SHAOLIN STAFF—BASIC SEQUENCES	D0920
SHAOLIN WHITE CRANE GONG FU BASIC TRAINING—COURSES 1 & 2	D599
SHAOLIN WHITE CRANE GONG FU BASIC TRAINING—COURSES 3 & 4	D0784
SHUAI JIAO—KUNG FU WRESTLING	D1149
SIMPLE QIGONG EXERCISES FOR ARTHRITIS RELIEF	D0890
SIMPLE QIGONG EXERCISES FOR BACK PAIN RELIEF	D0883
SIMPLIFIED TAI CHI CHUAN—24 & 48 POSTURES	D0630
SUNRISE TAI CHI	D0274
SUNSET TAI CHI	D0760
SWORD—FUNDAMENTAL TRAINING	D1095
TAI CHI CONNECTIONS	D0444
TAI CHI ENERGY PATTERNS	D0525
TAI CHI FIGHTING SET	D0509
TAIJI BALL QIGONG—COURSES 1 & 2	D0517
TAIJI BALL QIGONG—COURSES 3 & 4	D0777
TAIJI CHIN NA—COURSES 1, 2, 3, & 4	D0463
TAIJI MARTIAL APPLICATIONS—37 POSTURES	D1057
TAIJI PUSHING HANDS—COURSES 1 & 2	D0495
TAIJI PUSHING HANDS—COURSES 3 & 4	D0681
TAIJI WRESTLING	D1064
TAIJI SABER	D1026
TAIJI & SHAOLIN STAFF—FUNDAMENTAL TRAINING	D0906
TAIJI YIN YANG STICKING HANDS	D1040
TAI CHI CHUAN CLASSICAL YANG STYLE	D645
TAIJI SWORD—CLASSICAL YANG STYLE	D0452
UNDERSTANDING QIGONG 1—WHAT IS QI? • HUMAN QI CIRCULATORY SYSTEM	D069X
UNDERSTANDING QIGONG 2—KEY POINTS • QIGONG BREATHING	D0418
UNDERSTANDING QIGONG 3—EMBRYONIC BREATHING	D0555
UNDERSTANDING QIGONG 4—FOUR SEASONS QIGONG	D0562
UNDERSTANDING QIGONG 5—SMALL CIRCULATION	D0753
UNDERSTANDING QIGONG 6—MARTIAL QIGONG BREATHING	D0913
WHITE CRANE HARD & SOFT QIGONG	D637
WUDANG SWORD	D1903
WUDANG KUNG FU—FUNDAMENTAL TRAINING	D1316
WUDANG TAIJIQUAN	D1217
XINGYIQUAN	D1200
YMAA 25 YEAR ANNIVERSARY DVD	D0708

more products available from . . .

YMAA Publication Center, Inc. 楊氏東方文化出版中心

1-800-669-8892 • info@ymaa.com • www.ymaa.com

Printed in the USA
CPSIA information can be obtained
at www.ICGtesting.com
JSHW060041150824
68134JS00028B/2591